MW01484411

What People Are Saying About this Book . . .

"This book helped me see the message and direction the Commandments offer for me, and my life, and it was comforting, loving, incredible, really. I can honestly say that I want God's blessings upon me."

—**Robbie Davis, 16**

"Too many people worry about the Ten Commandments hanging on a wall, when the real issue is having them alive in our hearts. This book gives blood, pulse and soul to those rules to live by."

—**Terry Pluto,** author and columnist,
Akron Beacon Journal

"This book makes the Commandments come alive in a remarkable way so we can take a thorough inventory of our lives."

—**Pat Williams,** Senior VP, Orlando Magic
and author, *How to Be Like Jesus*

"This book will help you understand the simple abundance in the Commandments—time-honored laws, perfectly formulated common sense, a plan for living a happy, productive and principle-centered life. I recommend this incredibly loving book as a gift to someone you love and care about because we do not 'break' the Ten Commandments, rather, we can become 'broken' if we do not follow their God-given wisdom."

—**Linda Fuller cofounder,**
Habitat for Humanity International

"We must talk about the Commandments and what they mean for our lives. This excellent and very thorough book can help families do that. Hanging the Ten Commandments on the wall may be symbolically important, but how a family lives them is much more crucial."

—**Nancy Rivard,**
Founder, Airline Ambassadors

"This book makes the Commandments come alive for you and helps you see how important each one is to your day-by-day happiness and, become all that you were meant to be! Best of all, it will have a lasting positive impact on your life and for those with whom you share it."

—Rev. Dr. Robert A. Schuller, Pastor
Donna M. Schuller,
Crystal Cathedral

"This book is about the Commandments and God's intent behind each law, and the precise ways it applies to your everyday life. As you'll discover in each Commandment, God reveals something that is very important to your welfare. As you will read in this most important book by authors you've come to love and trust, you'll uncover what each one is and see how it brings truth and light to your life. May you find true joy in the blessings of God as you journey through each of these God-inspired chapters.

—Michael Pichette,
educator, Santa Fe Christian Schools
and author, *The Great Bundingle Race*

THE 10 COMMANDMENTS AND THE SECRET EACH ONE GUARDS–FOR YOU

Bettie B. Youngs, Ph.D., Ed.D. • Jennifer Leigh Youngs, A.A.

from the SMART TEENS—SMART CHOICES series

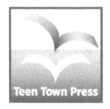

Teen Town Press
www.TeenTownPress.com

an imprint of Bettie Youngs Books

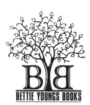

©2019 Bettie B. Youngs, Ph.D., Ed.D.; Jennifer Leigh Youngs, A.A.

All rights reserved. Printed in the United States of America. No part of this publication may be reproduced, stored in a retrieval system or transmitted in any form or by any means, electronic, mechanical, photocopying, recording or otherwise without the written permission of the publisher.

All Scripture quotations, unless otherwise indicated, are taken from the Holy Bible, New International Version® (NIV®). Copyright 1973, 1978, 1984 by International Bible Society. Used by permission of Zondervan Publishing House. Scriptures also from the New American Standard Bible, ©1960, 1962, 1963, 1968, 1971, 1972, 1973, 1975, 1977 by The Lockman Foundation. Used by permission. Other Scriptures from the King James Version, by permission. Also by permission HCI, original text, first printing; the pieces penned anonymously, are public domain, or contributed by teens.

Cover Graphic Design: Adrian Pitariu and Jane Hagaman
Text Design: Jane Hagaman
Editorial Consultant: Gerald L. Kuiper
Teen Consultant: Kendahl Brooke Youngs

TEEN TOWN PRESS / www.TeenTownPress.com is an Imprint of Bettie Youngs Book Publishing Co., Inc.:
www.BettieYoungsBooks.com; info@BettieYoungsBooks.com.

If you are unable to order this book from your local bookseller or online, you may order directly from the publisher:
info@BettieYoungsBooks.com.

ISBN: 978-1-940784-95-3 (trade paper)
ISBN: 978-1-940784-94-6 (e-book)

10 9 8 7 6 5 4 3 2

Library of Congress Cataloging-in-Publication Data Available upon Request.
Youngs, Bettie Burres.
FOR TEENS & YOUNG ADULTS: The 10 Commandments and the Secret Each One Guards—FOR YOU
Summary: Looks at how the Ten Commandments guides daily life for living a Christian life.
1. 10 Commandments—YA literature. 2. Christian Youth—Religious life—Juvenile literature. [1. Ten Commandments. 2. Christian life. 3. Daily Living. 4. Bettie Youngs, Ph.D., Ed.D.]

He who has my Commandments and keeps them,
it is he who loves Me.

John 14:21

A Special Word from the Authors

For the sake of simplicity and clarity, personal pronoun references to God in this book will be capitalized (i.e., He) while references to the person of Jesus Christ will be lowercased (he). This in no way makes a doctrinal statement but serves to make clear the distinction between the two entities.

Also by the Authors for Teens and Young Adults

FOR TEENS & YOUNG ADULTS: 12 Months of Faith: A Devotional Journal for Teens

FOR TEENS & YOUNG ADULTS: A Teen's Guide to Christian Living: Practical Answers to Tough Questions About God and Faith

FOR TEENS & YOUNG ADULTS: How Your Brain Decides If You Will Become Addicted—Or Not

FOR TEENS & YOUNG ADULTS: Setting and Achieving Goals That Matter—TO ME

FOR TEENS & YOUNG ADULTS: The Power of Being Kind, Courteous and Thoughtful

FOR TEENS & YOUNG ADULTS: How to Be Courageous

FOR TEENS & YOUNG ADULTS: How to Have a Great Attitude

FOR TEENS & YOUNG ADULTS: Growing Your Confidence and Self-Esteem

FOR TEENS & YOUNG ADULTS: Managing Stress, Pressure and the Ups and Downs of Life

FOR TEENS & YOUNG ADULTS: Caring for Your Body's Health and Wellness

FOR TEENS & YOUNG ADULTS: Having Healthy and Beautiful Hair, Skin and Nails

FOR TEENS & YOUNG ADULTS: 365 Days of Inspiration

FOR TEENS & YOUNG ADULTS: Inspirational Stories and Encouragement on Friends and the Face in the Mirror

FOR TEENS & YOUNG ADULTS: Inspirational Short Stories and Encouragement on Life, Love, and Issues

FOR TEENS & YOUNG ADULTS: My Journal on Life, Love and Making a Difference

CONTENTS

1

GOD'S TEN COMMANDMENTS—AND YOU

I have set My rainbow in the clouds, and it will be the sign of
the covenant between Me and the Earth.

Gen. 9:13

With love and honor, we welcome you to this book, an explo-
ration of the Ten Commandments and their relevance for you, a
young adult living in a time of unprecedented world events. What
exciting times! History is in the making, and you're a big part of
it. This is a time when you have more individual rights than ever
before, yet a time in which the preservation of those rights is at
risk. Many of your brothers and sisters the world over have yet to
have the oppressions from which they suffer lifted from their shoulders so that they, too, may rightfully lay claim to the freedoms you
enjoy, such as religious worship, safety and wellness, or a chance
to go about their lives with full opportunities for supporting their
families and enjoying their cultural heritage. May we each make it
our obligation, and our honor, to always look out for the welfare
of others and to safeguard their rights, just as we would our own.
Looking out for others—seeing our brothers and sisters through
the eyes of love—is at the heart of God's love.

Writing this book is such a privilege. In these pages, you'll get
a chance to explore a topic that is also about "safe-guarding welfare"—specifically your own—and discover how you can best provide leadership in these history-making times to which you've been
born. Throughout these pages, you'll take a walk through each of

the Ten Commandments—laws "inscribed by the finger of God" (Exod. 31:18)—and learn why and how each Commandment specifically guards something that is of the greatest importance to the welfare of every individual. What a paradise we could create here on Earth if we each would do our part.

We're all here for just a short time, really, although the mission we're on is huge. Contrary to our thinking that the world is a big place, it isn't. We can circle it within a day, and we can talk to practically anyone at any time of day or night. The world-place is, as my friend and astronaut Steve Smith describes, "a little planet that from space looks like a tiny blue marble laying on a Band-Aid-sized strip of black felt." Small or not, we're all here—and here for a reason. The mystery of it all unfolds in the laws inscribed by God, a covenant entered into between God and His people nearly 4,000 years ago.

Do you know the Commandments? Maybe your parents taught them to you as a young child, or you learned them in Sunday school. Maybe this is your first introduction. Or maybe you have some background but want to become more spiritually aware. This book will help you better understand God's love behind each of His Laws and discern how each applies to your everyday experiences.

Love of God and love for others are at the core of God's laws.

WHAT DO THE COMMANDMENTS MEAN TO YOU?

What do these ancient biblical laws mean to you, a young person living in exciting, yet turbulent, times? Do you think of the Commandments as old and outdated, or do you see them as incredibly pertinent? How do the Commandments serve you daily—from the moment you get out of bed, until your jam-packed and stress-filled day of dealing with others and fulfilling your obligations and responsibilities is over? How do the Commandments apply to the real-life issues young people face, such as a relationship with a special someone, or getting along with family members, friends, educators, employers and others you meet and greet throughout your day? How do the Commandments provide direction for the decisions you face and define the boundaries for your choices—such as staying healthy and fit, choosing or losing friends, attending college, choosing a career or setting goals for your future? How do the Commandments support you in coping with the problems in life, such as success, stress, depression, illness or debt? How do the Commandments both motivate and sustain you in times of crisis—such as the loss of a loved one, a personal setback, or confronting a disability, even a terminal illness? These are important questions, to be sure.

So, do these ancient laws—written 4,000 years ago—speak to you, a young adult living in today's time? You bet! This is a time in life in which you are discovering who you are and where you fit in. You're making important decisions about a lot of things. For example, you're willing to learn and follow the "rules" to be accepted and fit with your peers, but you also know just how much you will, or won't compromise to stay true to yourself. You're busy uncovering your strengths, talents and interests, knowing how important these are to your being all you can be.

The "Old" Commandments: Still Relevant Today

Up to now, you've been part of a "home family," and while that will always remain your "roots," you're finding your "wings" and discovering just how high and far you can fly. You naturally feel hopeful, optimistic and invincible. If you didn't feel this way, you might never venture into the world, where it awaits, even depends upon, your goodwill, your love, your youthful strength and energy, and most of all, your help and support—and your love of God.

Life is unfolding for you and you're seeing yourself as not just a bystander in life, but as an active participant and a leader. This, too, is a reason you will want to understand the laws—governed by love to God and to our neighbor—and see why God shines a spotlight on showing you the way to a meaning-filled and happy life, one that is strong and victorious.

Even though God gave the Ten Commandments thousands of years ago, they're still relevant. The need for safety, shelter and emotional security are still primary concerns in daily living; we still call upon God for guidance and direction as we maneuver through life and negotiate its challenges, frustrations and temptations. Throughout it all, we still can know where "the hand of God is that we might know how to live according to His will."

Why Did God Enter into a Covenant with His People?

At Mount Sinai (you'll get an overview of what happened there in the next chapter), God entered into a covenant with His people of Israel. A covenant is a contract that guarantees the fulfillment of what has been promised. You're probably familiar with the covenant God made with Noah. He put the rainbow in the sky as a sign that if Noah would build the ark and do all that God asked of him, then God would never again send a flood to destroy the Earth: "This is the sign of the covenant which I make between Me and you, and every living creature that is with you, for perpetual generations: I set My rainbow in the cloud, and it shall be for the sign of the covenant between Me and the Earth. It shall be when I bring a cloud over the Earth, that the rainbow shall be seen in the cloud" (Gen. 9:12–14 NKJV). Imagine, the beautiful rainbow comes to us as a promise of protection from our Heavenly Father—how totally cool is that?

At Mount Sinai, God pledged to make the Israelites a holy people whom He would use to bring salvation to all mankind. As a sign of acceptance and in celebration, Moses sacrificed an ox to the Lord, taking its blood and sprinkling it upon the altar (called "the blood of the covenant"). The people pledged to trust God and keep His word: "We will do everything the Lord has said; we will obey" (Exod. 24:7). As a sign of "sealing" the covenant, Moses said, "This is the blood of the covenant that the Lord has made with you in accordance with all these words" (Exod. 24:8).

If we ask what moved God to enter into a covenant with His people, there is only one answer: His love. He created us. We are made in His image. We are His heirs. To God, each life—each soul—has eternal value. Because of His love for us, He teaches us how to live a godly life. When we transgress—when we mess up or go astray—

He offers us forgiveness of sin through the Savior, and He leads us to faith in Jesus Christ that we might know eternal life. We are His children. He wants us to return to Him, to live with Him eternally. But God must live in us before He can work through us.

The love that moved God to give us the gospel also moved Him to give us His holy law. God first inscribed His law in the heart of man at creation; later He gave the Ten Commandments at Mount Sinai. We call the law inscribed in our hearts the conscience. "The Gentiles . . . show the work of the law written in their hearts, their conscience also bearing witness" (Rom. 2:14–15 KJV). The conscience is always on the side of what we believe to be right. Unless instructed by the Word of God, the conscience may be on the side of what is wrong because we believe it to be right. In order that we may know what is right, God has given us the written law.

The Commandments—Two Tablets "Inscribed by the Finger of God"

The Bible says that the Commandments were chiseled on the front and back of two stone tablets by God's own hand, "inscribed by the finger of God" (Exod. 31:18). Jesus divided the law into two parts—love for God and love for other people. The first four Commandments teach about love for God, and the last six Commandments address love for our neighbor. In the New Testament, when Jesus is asked which law is most important, he sums them all up into two parts, "Love the Lord thy God with all thy heart, and with all thy soul, and with all thy mind. This is the great and first Commandment. And the second is like unto it, thou shalt love thy neighbor as thyself" (Matt. 22:37–39 KJV).

As we learn in Romans 13:10, "Love is the fulfillment of the law." The purpose of the law is threefold:

> **To teach His people how to live.** "The Commandment is a lamp; and the law is light" (Prov. 6:23 KJV). We're born here on Earth, but we're not without direction on how to live here. Through the word of His Commandments, our

Heavenly Father takes us by the hand, inviting us to walk through life together with Him.

To teach us that we are not perfect—we sin. Yes, we try to be good and decent people, but our hearts are not as pure as God would like. The Commandments provide the baseline for what is "perfect," and so by comparing ourselves against each standard (i.e., "do not steal"), we know where we stand in God's eyes. If we are off base, our conscience accuses us and we know we've done wrong. "Through the law comes knowledge of sin" (Rom. 3:20 RSV).

To direct us to Christ. When we realize we have much to do in perfecting our nature, we try to do better. But even when we put all our willpower into the task of improving ourselves, we will be unable to produce the purity of heart that God asks of us in His law. Only forgiveness can bring peace to our conscience. Forgiveness of sin is the gift of Jesus Christ. "The law was put in charge to lead us to Christ" (Gal. 3:24).

In Each Commandment, God Guards Something that Is of Great Importance to Our Welfare

In much the same way that a loving parent provides rules to look after the safety and happiness of his child, so does our loving Heavenly Father provide rules—laws—for His people. To this end, the Commandments are loving, not limiting. In each Commandment, God guards something that is of the greatest importance to our welfare. Because each is a guideline for the way we should live, each address what we MUST do and MUST NOT do.

Each Commandment then, is a blueprint, a cornerstone used to govern our behavior. Even aside from the spiritual aspect, each is perfectly formulated "common sense," directing us to live in peace, harmony and safety with each other. They are the basis for moral and spiritual conduct, as well as the foundation of peace and prosperity for the individual and for the entire world, both then and now—and for always.

Can You Recite the Ten Commandments from Memory?

How familiar are you with the Ten Commandments? Can you recite them from memory? Throughout the coming chapters you'll get a chance to examine each of the Commandments in depth, but here they are, listed in the order in which God delivered them to us.

GOD'S TEN COMMANDMENTS (EXOD. 20:1–17)

1. I am the Lord your God. You shall have no other gods before me.
2. You shall not make for yourself an idol in the form of anything in heaven above or on the Earth beneath or in the waters below.
3. You shall not misuse the name of the Lord your God, for the Lord will not hold anyone guiltless who misuses his name.
4. Remember the Sabbath day by keeping it holy.
5. Honor your father and your mother so that you may live long in the land the Lord your God is giving you.
6. You shall not murder.
7. You shall not commit adultery.
8. You shall not steal.
9. You shall not give false testimony against your neighbor.
10. You shall not covet your neighbor's house, his wife, or his servant, his ox or donkey, or anything that belongs to your neighbor.

The Ten Commandments show us the way—still.

SIMPLE LOVE

We make His love too narrow
By false limits of our own,
We magnify His strictness
With a zeal He would not own.
If our love were but more simple
If we took Him at His Word,
Then our lives would be less complicated
And we'd know the sweetness of our Lord.

—Arlene Bernice Marion Burres

2

MOUNT SINAI: WHAT HAPPENED ON THE MOUNTAIN

... I carried you on eagles' wings ...

Exod. 19:4

When you think about the Ten Commandments, what's the first thing that comes to mind? Is it the movie with the commanding image of actor Charleton Heston as Moses, parting the Red Sea or holding the emblazoned stone tablets high above his head? It's an exciting movie to be sure, and it characterizes a good bit of the amazing history surrounding this most defining moment in time. Still, if you haven't already done so, you'll want to read Exodus 20 for yourself so that you get the full story!

MOUNT SINAI AND THE TEN COMMANDMENTS

You'll read that it was up on Mt. Sinai that God gave the Ten Commandments to Moses. But to better understand the gravity of what happened at Mount Sinai, it's important to know what events led up to it. The Israelites had been taken into slavery in Egypt, and God called a man named Moses to deliver them—to bring them out. God empowered Moses to stand against the Pharaoh (Ramses II), and He sent plagues upon Egypt to convince Pharaoh that he must allow God's people to leave. When the Israelites finally were given permission to leave and had started on their journey, the Egyptians changed their minds and gave chase. That's when the incredible event of the parting of the Red Sea took place. The Israelites walked through the sea on dry ground and then, when the Egyptians got into the riverbed, the invisible dam broke and the Egyptians drowned.

You'd think the Israelites would have been so awestruck by what God did that they'd live the rest of their lives in joyous thanksgiving, but not so. They got out into the desert and complained; they wanted to go back to Egypt because there they had food. God gave them fresh, heavenly food (manna) every morning. But when they grew tired of the manna, they complained again.

Three months after they left Egypt, they arrived at Mount Sinai. God told Moses to tell the people: "You yourselves have seen what I did to Egypt and how I carried you on eagles' wings and brought you to Myself. Now if you obey Me fully and keep My covenant, then out of all nations you will be My treasured possession" (Exod. 19:4–5). God also told Moses that in three days He would come to the top of the mountain and the people should be ready. At the appointed time, God arrived with thunder, lightning, a trumpet blast that grew louder and louder, and a cloud of smoke that covered and billowed off the top of Mount Sinai like a furnace. The mountain trembled, and so did the Israelites! It must have been spectacular!

24/7—Forty Days . . . and Forty Nights!

Moses then went up on the mountain as God instructed and stayed for forty days and forty nights. While he was there, God inscribed the Ten Commandments. The Bible says that the Commandments were chiseled on the front and back of two stone tablets by God's own hand—"inscribed by the finger of God" (Exod. 31:18). God gave the Commandments so He could enter into this covenant with the Israelites. A covenant is a contract that guarantees the fulfillment of what has been promised.

At Mount Sinai, God entered into a covenant with His people of Israel. He pledged Himself to be their God and to make them a holy people whom He would use to bring salvation to all mankind. As a sign of acceptance and celebration, Moses sacrificed an ox to

God, taking its blood and sprinkling it upon an altar. This covenant sealed with blood is called the "blood of the covenant." The people pledged themselves to trust God and keep His word: "All that the Lord has said we will do, and be obedient" (Exod. 24:3–8). As a sign of "sealing" the covenant, Moses said, "This is the blood of the covenant which the Lord has made with you according to all these words" (Exod. 24:8).

An Outraged Moses Break the Tablets . . .
and God Calls Him Back

Meanwhile, at the foot of the mountain, the Israelites already were abandoning God. They gathered all their gold, melted it down and created a calf—to which they bowed down and worshipped. Can you believe their foolishness? Understandably, when Moses came down off the mountain carrying the tablets, he was so outraged that he threw the tablets down and broke them. Then God called Moses back to the mountain. It's hard to tell who was more angry, God or Moses, but Moses pleaded with God to give the people another chance.

God said to Moses, "The Lord, the compassionate and gracious God, slow to anger, abounding in love, and faithfulness, maintaining love to thousands, and forgiving wickedness, rebellion, and sin. I am making a covenant with you" (Exod. 34:6–7, 10). God forgave the people for abandoning him and again chiseled the Ten Commandments on two new stone tablets. "When Moses came down from Mount Sinai with the two tablets of the Testimony in his hands . . . his face was radiant because he had spoken with the Lord" (Exod. 34:29). At first, seeing the radiance, the people were afraid of Moses, but when he reassured them, they came to him and he gave them the covenant that God had established.

A Chest Lined with Gold to Store the Stone Tablets

After Moses gave God's message to the people, he built a wooden chest overlaid and lined with gold—as per God's specific instructions (Exod. 25:10–22)—and placed the tablets in this chest.

Because the Israelites had not yet claimed the land that God had promised them, they carried the precious box with them wherever they went. They called the chest and tablets the Ark of the Covenant or the Ark of the Testimony because it represented God's covenant to be their God and His promise to dwell with them.

What Happened to the Tablets After Mount Sinai?

Did you ever wonder what happened to the tablets after the Israelites left Mt. Sinai? It's a fascinating story. Because God had made the importance of the Ark of the Covenant very clear to them, the people treasured and protected the Ark above everything and everyone; it was a symbol that God was God and that He was watching over them. Even other people knew that God's glory dwelt in the Ark, and the inevitable happened. Another tribe stole the Ark of the Covenant, but they didn't get the results they had hoped for (1 Sam. 4–5)!

The Philistines overthrew the Israelites and captured the Ark of the Covenant. Thinking they had the ultimate power, they took the gold-lined chest bearing the tablets to their temple and placed it beside the statue of their god Dagon. The next morning Dagon was facedown! The Philistines righted the worthless statue only to find it again facedown and broken the next morning. But their trouble was just beginning. Next, the people of Ashdod were afflicted with tumors, so, not surprisingly, the leaders had a meeting. They decided that having the Lord's Ark wasn't a good thing, so they unloaded it by moving it to Gath.

The Lord's hand was heavy on them, as well, and the people of that city, both young and old, were also afflicted with an outbreak of tumors. The people of Gath moved the Ark to a third city. The people of Ekron fared no better. They already had heard the rumors of the troubles the other towns had endured when in possession of the golden chest and weren't at all happy to see the Ark of the Covenant coming their way. God was consistent; many people in Ekron died, and the rest were afflicted with, you guessed it, tumors and destruction. Not surprisingly, the Philistines were beginning to get the picture that the God of Israel was thoroughly ticked-off that they had stolen His Ark!

The Trick That Didn't Work Out . . .

The Philistines devised a little experiment. They placed the Ark on a cart drawn by two oxen and sent it toward the Israelite camp. Complicating the experiment, each of the oxen had a calf that the Philistines locked up. Because it's completely abnormal for a mother ox to deliberately walk away from her offspring, they would know that the God of Israel was, indeed, the one and only God if the oxen went against all nature and traveled with the Ark away from their calves.

Imagine the Philistines standing by the road and watching expectantly as they put their experiment into motion. The oxen traveled straight for the Israelite camp and never looked back. The Israelites were thrilled beyond measure to have their beloved Ark returned, and the Philistines were just as happy to be rid of it! It just goes to show that God was obviously very protective of His stone tablets bearing His Ten Commandments. They were the representation of His covenant with His people, and no one was going to change the plan.

The Ark of the Covenant (Here's Where Indiana Jones Fits into All This)

When the Israelites built the temple in Jerusalem, the gold-lined chest holding the precious stone tablets was placed in the inner sanctum, the most holy place in the temple. It was called the Holy of Holies because God's presence and glory dwelt in that place. On penalty of death, no one could enter except the high priest who went in once a year to offer sacrifices for the atonement of sins. The Ark of the Covenant was there in the Holy of Holies until the Babylonians destroyed the temple in 586 BC. After that, the Ark of the Covenant disappeared and, to this day, its whereabouts is a mystery. Obviously, there is much speculation among scientists, archeologists and historians as to what happened to the beautiful chest. Many think it may still be buried under the foundation of what once was the temple (under what is now the Muslim-controlled Dome of the Rock), but so far, it has not been uncovered. Does this all sound a little familiar? Maybe you know the Bible story, or maybe you saw Indiana Jones looking for the Ark of the Covenant in the movie *Indiana Jones and the Last Crusade*. Hollywood theatrics aside, it's a fascinating thought that the Ark may still exist, isn't it?

This, of course, is just a thumbnail sketch of the history of the amazing tablets. You can read the Book of Exodus and 1 Samuel 4–6 to get the whole story. One thing is for sure, you'll not find a story anywhere half as interesting!

The actual tablets have disappeared, but their message is still the cornerstone of human civilization. Simply amazing.

Ancient Freedom

To live a life of joy and freedom,
It's the Commandments you must obey.
They're so much more than ancient words,
They're the rules for work and play.

To live a life of joy and freedom,
Let God walk with you throughout your day.
Then relationships become a privilege
Because you've allowed your will His way.

To live a life of joy and freedom,
When challenging times lead you astray,
Know that Jesus knows your struggles,
Just call on him, listen, read and pray.

To live a life of joy and freedom,
Dare to go beyond what others say.
Yes, it takes courage to live beyond the limits,
Do you really want it any other way?

—Mandy Pohja, 17

3

THE FIRST COMMANDMENT

I am the Lord your God. You shall have no other gods before me.

Exod. 20:2–3

In the previous section you reviewed the events leading up to the historically monumental "inauguration" of the Commandments. In a most spectacular display of dramatics (which to date, no rock group has been able to upstage!), God "descended to the top of Mount Sinai and called Moses to the top of the mountain. Moses went up" (Exod. 19:20). The rest is history: Moses went up on the mountain where God gave him the Ten Commandments—His laws for moral and spiritual conduct and the foundation for peace and prosperity for His children. The Scripture goes like this: "When the Lord finished speaking to Moses on Mount Sinai, He gave him the two tablets of the Testimony, the tablets of stone inscribed by the finger of God" (Exod. 31:18). What a beautifully touching image!

In a nutshell, the Commandments are a covenant, an agreement, basically saying, "My part is that I'll be your God and I'll take care of you and provide direction as to how you must conduct yourselves—in mind, body and spirit—down here on Earth (via the Commandments). Your part is to live according to these laws, which are essentially governed by love for God and love for your neighbor."

So that we might know, trust and listen to this direction, God establishes His leadership right off the bat. In the first Commandment, we learn exactly WHO oversees things. God starts by introducing himself, "I am the Lord your God" and then issues this foreboding command: "You shall have no other gods before me." In this powerful first law, God establishes right up front that HE—and only He—is God. Not only is He God, but He is our God, and we are to put Him first and foremost in our lives. We are to revere, love and trust Him above all things.

In each of His Commandments, God guards something that is of supreme importance to our lives. In this Commandment, God is guarding the single most important prized possession we humans ever will have: God's love. The first Commandment, then, reassures us there is One on High, an almighty and omnipotent force—God—whose love for us is beyond any kind of love and magnificence we humans can possibly imagine. It outshines and outlasts any love we ever could hope to have here on Earth, including the abiding and unconditional lifelong love of our parents, or the romantic and serving love of a soul mate by our side throughout our lives. God's love is far greater than love we will experience here on Earth, even though some people here will love us dearly. What an awesome knowing!

God is revere-worthy, love-worthy and trust-worthy. Upholding the first Commandment shows that we revere, love and trust God, and love our "neighbors" as God loves us.

GOD'S FIRST COMMANDMENT IS RELEVANT TODAY

Much like we study for a driver's test to understand road safety, or review classroom rules on the first day of school, rules are necessary for the benefit of all. That Commandments were needed in ancient times to teach everyone the rules—we can see the logic in that. That in the beginning God would need to teach everyone about Himself—"I am the Creator, Master of the Universe, and your Heavenly Father"—is also reasonable. The first Commandment was relevant then.

But that was then, and this is now, right? The Bible and God's

Word have been around for nearly 4,000 years. Christianity has withstood the test of time. We know there is a God (even if He is defined and described in different ways). How, then, does the first Commandment speak to us today—when millions of people haven't figured out how to live in peace?

God knew that our lives would be a battlefield of challenges, but He also knew our hearts. We are made to love God, and we must remember that we were created because of God's love. God speaks to us in our hearts and listens to our hearts. He knows that it is in the heart where battles are won and lost. God wants us to find our way to Him, which is why He created a longing for Him in our hearts. We each have a mission, a divine purpose for our lives.

And just what might that be? An important premise, one that we Christians believe with all our hearts, is that there is a reason for our being. This ideal is rooted in faith, felt in our hearts, expressed in our joy and lived in our actions daily.

Is There a Divine Purpose for Your Life?

What do you think is the purpose of your life? Is it to clean your room, go to school, get your homework done, go to church, go to college, get a job, get married, raise a family, go to work daily, and then retire? And then what? Is the purpose of our lives about the roles we create for ourselves and then go about fulfilling? Or is there more? The Bible tells us we are made in God's image. If your birthright is that of an heir, you're in God's family—which means you have a legacy to fulfill. Do you believe that your life has the divine purpose of being an heir to God's kingdom—or that it has not much more intention than, say, a blade of grass or a mushroom?

For Christians the answer is simple and straightforward: We are on a journey. We are trying to find our way home. Home to God. We want eternal life with our Father, our Heavenly Father, our Creator. How do we get there? Figuratively and literally, we are to follow the map we'll find in God's "textbook" for the great school of life (the Bible). Here we will find clear and concise directions (the

Commandments) for how to live our lives God's way. The Commandments are God's "streetlight" for us to follow; they are God's "rules" for our play and for our work. The Commandments give the answers to the battlefield of challenges we all face in our lives—and in them we find eternal life.

Are You on a Journey—or Chasing After the Wind?

Would you characterize your life as routine, too busy, even boring? Do you feel tired and drained, as though you need to "get a life"? That can happen, especially if we lose sight of the reason why we're here, the reason we have life in the first place. Hopefully, you believe it is your "earthly work" to be filled with His Holy Spirit, and all services and duties rendered in your life-time are a "reasonable response" to being loved by God. If so, then your life has meaning, purpose and direction. Are you following God's spotlight shining the way to a glorious life that is pure, strong and victorious? That is the reason for the journey. But what if we get lost or detoured along the way—what if "life happens"?

The Commandments offer direction. God does not put us here on this Earth and say, "There you go. Have a nice trip. Hope to see you later." We need to be instructed on how "life works." God knows this. The Commandments offer the guidelines for how "life works," starting off with the assurance we find in the first Commandment in which God basically says, "Listen to My voice, that you might know Me. Listen to My guidance, that you might learn how to walk. Feel My love, that you might truly love yourself and others. Hear My Word, that you might share it with your siblings—all over the Earth. I'm here for you—call on Me. I am the Lord your God."

God sets about parenting us. He directs that a relationship with Him is to be the focus, in fact, the very core of our lives. We are to be firmly rooted in God. The command is clear: God is to be #1 in our lives—all the time and in all ways. Scripture tells us that we are not to place concern for livelihood before Him, nor the acquisition of money or material possessions, not fame or popularity—or anything else. Why? Because "chasing" after these things would serve only to separate us from God, and God knows no amount of "stuff" can bring us happiness. As we learn in Ecclesiastes 2:4–17 (RSV): "I made great works; I built houses and vineyards for myself. I bought male and female slaves. . . . I had also great herds and flocks. . .. I also gathered for myself silver and gold and the treasures of kings. . .. I kept my heart from no pleasure. Then I considered all that my hands had done and the toil I had spent doing it all was vanity and a striving after wind. . . . So, I hated life for all is vanity and a striving after wind."

Do You Place God First and Foremost in Your Life?

Our Heavenly Father knows us—after all, He made us—and He knows there is only one thing that satisfies our soul: living according to His commandments. All else is fleeting: "Naked a man comes from his mother's womb, and as he comes, so he departs" (Eccles. 5:15). We are to do as Jesus said, "Worship the Lord your God, and serve Him only" (Matt. 4:10). We must not idolize anything that detracts us from the purpose of our earthly journey, which is to experience God's love and know His will. If our lives are to have meaning at all, if they are to serve any purpose, then we must live according to the Commandments. But God must live in us before He can work through us.

The first Commandment begins with God's instructions as to what we are to do and not to do to be "heirs" to God. Because we are grateful for this guidance that leads to the path of eternal life, we naturally should revere, love and trust God. Revere, love and trust: What do these terms really mean?

WHAT DOES IT MEAN TO "REVERE" GOD?

We are to revere God. In many instances the Bible says we are to "fear" God. When God speaks about a consequence for not following a command, there is no doubt about the authoritative voice with which He speaks. Does the notion "to fear God" make God seem a little foreboding? We'd rather think of God as loving and forgiving, but the truth is, we'd better fear Him as well. Consider His words, ". . . I, the Lord your God, am a jealous God, punishing the children for the sin of the fathers to the third and fourth generation of those who hate Me . . ." (Exod. 20:5). If that doesn't make anyone quake, what will? Thankfully, He follows these very words with, ". . . but showing love to a thousand (generations) of those who love Me and keep My commandments" (Exod. 20:6).

To "revere" God means to stand in awe of His power, His authority, His greatness. Jesus said, "All authority in heaven and on Earth has been given to me" (Matt. 28:18). Therefore, to fear God means to acknowledge His authority and to revere His position as the one and only God.

What Would You Think, Do or Say if God Dropped In on You?

To help you get a sense for the "reverence" we're to have for God, place Him in your presence for a moment. Imagine that God has, without notice, joined you and your family at the dinner table. Or He's decided to pop in at your school and greets you at your locker or takes a seat next to you at lunch. Or maybe He decides to join you at your job and meets up with you by the watercooler. Approaching you He says in a loving, but most unyielding voice, "Hi. I am the Lord your God, and you're to have no other gods before me." How would you feel? This is God, your Creator. Your Heavenly Father. The one who knew you "even as you were knit together in your mother's womb" (from Ps. 139:13), the One who sits in charge come Judgment Day.

Think back to a time when a teacher (or parent, coach or employer) called you on something because you'd been out of line. How did you feel? Did the fact that you'd been called on by a person in a position of authority get your attention? Did it make you a tad bit "fearful"? No doubt it did. Likewise, God wants us to revere Him, knowing that he is most serious about the Laws He's given us. Take a moment to reflect on God's command in His first law. Only a fool wouldn't "listen up," right? That's what reverence is—the kind of "fear" for which God is deserving. And by the way, the thought of God sitting near you at school or at work isn't all that farfetched because God is always that close to us—every day and in every way. Do all you can to be worthy of God's love.

God promises consequences for all who transgress against His commandments. We therefore should revere Him and not break His laws. As we learn in Galatians 6:7, "Do not be deceived; God cannot be mocked; a man reaps what he sows." But He promises grace and every blessing to all who keep His laws. We should therefore love Him and trust Him, and gladly keep His commandments. We find a fearful seriousness in what God says of sin: "The soul who sins is the one who will die" (Ezek. 18:4).

"Fearful Seriousness": God Does Not Shy Away from Reminding us of Consequences

God does not shy away from reminding us there are consequences for not obeying the laws He set forth to guide our lives in the direction of fulfilling our purpose. He doesn't just say, "These commandments are to help you live orderly lives and to be able to know what is expected of each person, but it's okay if you do your own thing." Nor does He say, "If some of you want to live by them, good. And if others refuse, that's okay, too."

What would life be like if each of us "did our own thing"— lived in the way we each simply chose to? Would the bullies of the world oppress the meek, timid and shy among us? God knows this and says that all the laws apply to each one of us. If we refuse to obey them, then consequences follow. We should take heed: The agony of an accusing conscience is one form of punishment. Loss of honor, health, friends and property are other forms. Eternal separation from God is the last and worst punishment.

The Bible tells us that even the sins of the fathers come as punishment upon children who hate God. Parents' evil reputation, immorality and other forms of ungodliness are inherited and increased in children who continue in the same evil ways. Sin becomes a destructive curse from generation to generation. This is heavy and serious, isn't it? But on the flip side, consider that we also have God's blessings. God shows mercy to us in order to encourage, inspire and enable us to live according to His will. This is how much God loves His children and wants us to return to the fold. If we ask for forgiveness, God forgives. For even the most serious things that we do, if we repent (ask God to make us new, whole and pure), He wipes the slate clean. He then makes us a blessing to other people.

The Fear and Love of God Are the Strongest Building Forces in Human Life

God's love is so encompassing that when we ask Him into our lives, He uses our sufferings, our battlefield of challenges, as a means for building up our spiritual lives. Fear and love of God are the strongest building forces in human life, while sin is the greatest destroyer. "We know that to them that love God all things work together for good" (Rom. 8:28).

God's blessings do not stop with the individual; they are inherited by their children and shared by society. The human family is so closely knit together that we transmit to our children both the fruits of our sins and the blessings of a God-fearing life. "But from everlasting to everlasting, the Lord's love is with those who fear him, and his righteousness with their children's children" (Ps. 103:17). "Godliness has value for all things, holding promise for both the present life and the life to come" (1 Tim. 4:8).

The Commandments teach us how our Heavenly Father wants us to live. It is a beautiful life, pure, strong, victorious and governed by love to God and to our neighbor. As much as we'd like to think we're simply the best, we all sin and need forgiveness. God provided this forgiveness by sending His Son to die for us and by giving us His Holy Spirit. Is it difficult to accept that a God who grants us our lives and provides for us would not have stiff penalties for those who don't follow His laws? No. What is at stake when we disobey His commands? Nothing less than eternal life.

Revering, Loving and Trusting God

"I know teens who turn to God only when it's convenient for them, like when they're really hurting or stressed. I even know kids with an 'I am too cool to need God' attitude and so they roll their eyes when anyone talks about God. And, I know teens who think of God as everything is love, love, love. Having a relationship with God is a very different thing—the real thing." —Carren Amos, 17

"When I was little, I thought my parents were silly to make me get off my bike and look both ways before crossing the street, so when I thought they weren't looking, I'd glance both ways and ride on across. One day I rode out from behind a parked car into the path of a car. The driver braked and swerved, but he still clipped my bike. My leg was broken, and I spent months in a cast. God didn't break my leg because I disobeyed my parents, but I learned a valuable lesson. To me, that's what fearing the Lord means—to listen and respect. You know, cause, effect; it's a pretty simple equation." —Debbie Del Guercio, 13

"To me, what God expects is pretty clear: The commandments spell it all out. I like knowing I have God's guidance. It's amazing how simple and straight-forward life gets when I put God first." —Brad Tomelson, 16

WHAT DOES IT MEAN TO "LOVE" GOD?

God's love is so much higher and purer than any human love. God loved us when He created the world and then human beings to go in it. He loved us when Adam and Eve sinned, so He sent Jesus, his one and only Son, to demonstrate His love for us and to die on the cross to pay for our sins (John 3:16). Even then, God looked down through the ages and knew there would be a you and a me and even knew us by name. He saw us when we were formed in our mothers' womb (Isaiah 44:2) and knows us so well that He numbers every hair on our heads (Matthew 10:30). Now that is an amazing brand of love!

Let's back up and explore Jesus' role in God's love because it's pivotal in understanding just how much God loves us. Think for a moment about your life and the way you've been living it up to know. Now consider standing before God and answering for the choices you've made. But before you even do that, think about standing before a Judge in a Court of law. Consider for a moment, that you are standing before a judge with answering for a crime, an offense, you'd committed. The Judge is about to hand down your sentence. You probably quake at the prospect of the verdict you know you deserve. However, instead of reading you the sentence, then slamming down his gavel and dismissing you, the judge looks at you tenderly and says to you, "I consider you as my child, but you are free to go because someone else paid your penalty." That's the kind of judge God will be when you stand before Him to answer for the choices you've made in your life. That's how much God loves you and me. "This is love, not that we loved God, but that he loved us and sent his Son as an atoning sacrifice for our sin" (I John 4:10).

If you have accepted that Jesus traded places with you, then your sins are forgiven. God sees you as sinless as Jesus. That's what happened when He traded places with you. If that weren't enough, God gave you life and sustains it every day. The air you breathe, the food you eat, the clothes you wear, your family, your friends, your ability to learn—are all gifts from God because He loves you. Even if we think something is missing, perhaps your parents are separated or divorced and you don't get to spend as much time with one or both of them as you'd like, or making good grades doesn't come easily for you, or you're not as athletic as you'd like—God loves you as you as you are.

Allowing us to struggle is a part of God's love for us because our struggles make us stronger. God has a perfect plan for your life, and it doesn't look like anyone else's perfect plan. Yes, it's perfect—even though we look around and sometimes wonder why others have it "bigger, better, brighter." You didn't get gypped: Trust that God knows what He's doing. If you question any of this, have a heart to heart talk with God. Trust that God is wanting to hear from you.

You can understand the concept of divine love through experiencing unconditional love in your own home. Of course, not all of you have that kind of home, and when love is absent or dysfunctional, it becomes more difficult to identify with a loving God who cares the same for all of us, but who allows us to choose to love Him. God's love is not based on who we are, what kind of grades we make, how well we fit in or any of the other criteria against which young people sometime measure themselves. We're each uniquely made by God expressly for relationship with Him. That means He wants us to know Him intimately and to love Him because we desire that relationship more than anything. He loves us enough to wait for us to come to Him. He gently prods but gives us room to decide.

So, what do we do with so great a love? We return it: we follow the Commandments He set forth as a code of conduct; we align our will with His, and we trust and believe with all our hearts that God has a plan for our lives.

> *"I'm sure that God loves me. And, I trust that from this love He has a plan for me. I want my love of God to show up in all the things I do, from how I treat others, to bringing God into the decisions I make. I want to be a loving person."* —Brian Burres, 15

> *"God's love for me doesn't mean that He drops a cool convertible in my driveway or gives me the answers to an exam I didn't study for or makes all my problems go away. God's love for me means that He'll be by side as I walk through good times and bad. I'm closer to God and stronger as a result of having struggled with some things."* —Noah Johnson, 16

WHAT DOES IT MEAN TO "TRUST" GOD?

To be trusted is the highest compliment. Trust is an important quality and one for which the measuring stick is one we keep deep within our hearts. Who can you trust? For sure we can trust God as we learn in Psalms 84:1-2: *"Blessed is the man who trusts in the*

LORD, and whose hope is the LORD. For he shall be like a tree planted by the waters, which spreads out its roots by the river, and will not fear when heat comes; but its leaf will be green and will not be anxious in the year of drought, nor will cease from yielding fruit."

Trust means to depend on, to have faith in, confidence in, security in. A beautiful scripture is Proverbs 3:5–6: *"Trust in the Lord with all your heart and lean not on your own understanding. In all your ways acknowledge him, and he will make your paths straight."* Our mandate to trust God further clarifies that we not to "lean on our own understanding."

> *"I'm at a crossroads in my life right now. I've got lots of important decisions to make—where I'll go to college, what I will major in and what career that will lead to. I'm really in love with a guy and we're trying to decide if being engaged is the best and right decision, or not. I know that with the freedom of college we'll both have opportunities to be with others. I could be 'crazed' over it, but really, the best thing for me to do is to put my faith and trust in God and ask Him to watch over me, and the person I love. I trust that whatever happens, God considers it best and right for me."* —Kerri Mathis, 18

> *"When I find myself all anxious and apprehensive about things, I turn it over to God. I trust Him to help me handle things."* —Luke Ellis, 16

God is Revere-Worthy, Love-Worthy and Trust-Worthy

Put God first in your life. Talk with God daily about your joys, sadness, problems. Ask Him to help you have a glorious life, one that is pure, strong and victorious.

QUESTIONS FOR REFLECTION

- Do you consider God's love as the single most "prized possession" you have? In what way is having God's love a "blessing" to you?

- The first commandment reassures us that we are not without "leadership." Do you ever think of God in this way—as a leader? In what ways does God offer leadership to your life?

- The first commandment asks us to revere God. In what way do you consider God "revere-worthy"?

- Do you believe there is a purpose for your life, a reason for your being? If so, what is your purpose?

- How would others know you are a "God-centered" person?

- How would you react if God suddenly appeared at your side, such as when you were standing in line for the movies with your friends, or sat down beside you at lunch? Would it scare you, or would you feel humbled, honored and joyous to meet your Creator?

- *"Be not deceived; God is not mocked; for whatsoever a man sows, that shall he also reap"* [Galatians 6:7]. What does this Scripture mean to you? Has God ever given you a consequence for something you did? How do you know it was God who was levying the consequence? What did you do, and what was God's "consequence"?

- *"Trust in the Lord with all your heart and lean not on your own understanding. In all your ways acknowledge him, and he will make your paths straight"* [Proverbs 3:5-6]. What does this Scripture mean to you?

Angels in Our Midst

Angels on the subway
Angels in the park
Angels in a lighthouse
Angels guarding in the dark.

Angels in the taxi
Angels on the train
Angels walking down Main Street
Angels dancing in the rain.

Angels in the bakery
Angels packing bags to go to camp
Angels at the grocery store
Angels on the parking ramp.

Angels singing at a wedding
Angels walking down school halls
Angels playing professional soccer
Angels at the local mall.

Angels doing yoga
Angels teaching at your school
Angels taking photos
Angels swimming in the pool.

Angels working in the office
Angels writing spirit books
Angels cooking a favorite dinner
God's love . . . is everywhere you look!

—Stephanie Lloyd, 14

4

THE SECOND COMMANDMENT

"You shall not make for yourself an idol in the form of anything in heaven above or on the earth beneath or in the waters
below. You shall not bow down to them nor serve them."

Exod. 20:4-5

In the first Commandment God introduced Himself and
instructed us to place our love of Him above all things. Having
established this foundation, God then orders through the second
Commandment that we have but one God. We are explicitly for-
bidden to make or serve idols—of any kind—regardless of what we
find attractive, desirable or honorable in high or low places. We are
to pursue God with the clarity of single-minded focus.

As with all the Commandments, God guards something that is
of great importance to our welfare. In the previous Commandment
it was letting us know with total certainty that GOD IS GOD—the
real thing, the one and only. In this second Commandment, God
is guarding His relationship between Him and us—His children.
We are commanded NOT to place anything—figuratively or literally—before Him. Why? Because doing that would interfere with
our knowing and loving God in the way He intends. Anything that
comes between God and us could separate us from Him. If we place
the love of our parents, a boy- or girlfriend, brothers or sisters,
friends, the attainment of goals—or anything else—as more important than a relationship with Him, then we may never understand the

purpose of our lives, the "why-are-we-here" question, which Psalm 143:10a clarifies as: "Teach me to do your will, for you are my God." Obeying the second Commandment shows that we revere, love and trust God, and we love our "neighbors" as God loves us.

God is serious that we see this law as essential: After telling us that we must not bow down to idols or in any way serve them, God tells us the ramifications should we not heed his law: "I, the Lord your God, am a jealous God, punishing the children for the sin of the fathers to the third and fourth generation of those who hate Me" (Exod. 20:5). Yes, this sounds harsh. Many young adults reject this facet of God, but they shouldn't.

God does levy consequences for those who transgress His Commandments, and we therefore should have a serious fearfulness about upholding them. And remember this: God promises grace and every blessing to all who keep and uphold the Commandments. We therefore should love and trust Him, and gladly keep His Commandments. We find a fearful seriousness in what God says of the punishment of sin: "The soul who sins is the one who will die" (Ezek. 18:4). And in Galatians 6:7, "Do not be deceived; God cannot be mocked; a man reaps what he sows." God gives more space to this Commandment than to any of the others, so it must be important to Him. Therefore, we can assume that it better be important to us.

GOD'S SECOND COMMANDMENT IS STILL RELEVANT TODAY

In what ways does this ancient Commandment have relevancy for our lives today? In a time when "extreme" is the standard and "manifesting" is but a dial tone away, how can we keep God at the center of our lives and need Him more than anything or anyone else? Do we need to be concerned that in a time when anything and everything is within our reach—from fast food to fast cars; from Internet chat rooms to cell phones capable of taking and sending pictures; and, when travel options include reserving a seat on the next trip to the moon, that many of God's children would rather play with their "toys" than focus on the lesson in the second Commandment? From screen idols to American Idols to teen idols, can the second Commandment help us decide who is the best of the best, the winner, the "one and only"?

Are You "Good to Go" on the Second Commandment?

Do you think this Commandment has relevance in your life? Where is God on your list of priorities? In what ways do the things you desire and to which you aspire take priority over your time and need for God? Is God at the center of your life? Are there any "idols" in your life that move God out of His "Head Honcho" spot? Or maybe you feel as sixteen-year-old Colin Long does: "I'm 'good to go' on the second Commandment. I don't go around carving golden calves to worship; I don't belong to any cults." Is he "good to go"—or do you think God's intent behind His commandment requires more scrutiny?

God Knows Our Nature; He Knows
We Need Leadership and Inspiration

Why do you suspect God carefully and thoroughly clarifies His intent behind this second law? Maybe one reason is because God knows our nature—He knows that it is natural for us humans to desire (idolize) things. To get a sense of how easy we humans desire not just leadership but figureheads, imagine you are observing all that was taking place when Moses was up on Mount Sinai receiving the Ten Commandments. Because Moses had been gone so long, the Jewish people worried that maybe He wasn't returning: "We don't know what has happened to him," they said (Exod. 32:1). Then they said to Aaron (who was put in charge while Moses was away), "Come, make us gods who will go before us."

Aaron said to the people, "'Then break off your golden earrings from your wives, daughters and sons and bring them to me' . . . and he (Aaron) fashioned the gold into a molded calf, and they rose early on the next day, offered burnt offerings and brought peace offerings" (Exod. 32:2, 4, 6).

When God observed the Israelites making a golden calf, He was furious! "They have turned aside from what I commanded," God said to Moses. "They made an idol and worshiped it and sacrificed to it. My wrath burns hot against them and I may consume them" (Exod. 32:8, 10).

This shows that it's best not to mess with God! This is a good example of what we learned in the previous chapter, where you read that on some level we should "fear" God. God expects us to obey His laws. "I the Lord am a jealous God." Have you ever wondered what God means by that? As a teen, I wondered why God would be jealous of anything, especially when in this very Commandment He asks us not to be jealous of others nor of the things they have. But God wants us to obey His laws because He wants His children to return to Him. He is serious about spelling out what it is we are to do—and not do—that we might know life everlasting. Just as with our parents, there is much love behind the rules. Know the rules. And abide by them. Your life as a Christian is what this earthly journey is about.

To finish our story, Moses, duly afraid for his people, pleaded with God not to be angry. Mercifully (and just as you've probably experienced when your parents threatened to ground you for life—and didn't), God lets them off the hook: "Then the Lord relented and did not bring on His people the disaster He had threatened" (Exod. 32:14). What a loving Father!

What Does God Consider an "Idol"?

It is God's intent, then, that He be first in our minds, our hearts and our lives. Anything that crowds out our love for God as our first and primary mission in life is an "idol"—be it a person, money, position or power, and so on. Why would it be important for God to demand such total allegiance? Because when we put other things before our love of God, then it becomes impossible to live a holy life. Complacency, pride, greed, jealousy and fear, for example, keep us alienated from God. Thus, we are no longer "in relationship" with Him. We are no longer acting out His will; we are no longer on the mission of our lives—which is to be worthy of the journey home to God.

Perhaps we feel guiltless because we identify this concept with the Israelites who melted down their gold and created a golden calf. We consider ourselves far wiser than to do something like that! But even if we're not creating golden idols, we have our visual aids, too. It may be a person, such as an evangelist, a minister or youth pastor. As long it enriches our worship of God, this can be useful and valuable. However, the danger is in valuing the object or person too much so that it turns our focus away from God. Sometimes this is a subtle shift, and we may not notice it—unless and until the obvious hits us over the head! Sixteen-year-old Shannon Aldridge tells of an incident in which a "screaming heart" alerted her to this reality.

A year ago, I got involved in a youth group that met every Thursday evening right after school. The first couple of weeks I attended, I listened and took to heart the message of the importance of having a personal relationship with Jesus as a means of filling the void. God was my source of comfort and the reason I attended. By the third week I was even more interested in attending, but my reason for gladly going was a little different. The group leader was a twenty-four-year-old college student, someone I found extremely attractive. I think it would be safe to say I was falling in love. When I first started going, I sat in the very back row. By the third session, I was in the middle row. The fourth time, I was front and center! Halfway through the sessions, Mike left to attend a master's degree program in another state. He was replaced by a female graduate student. I was so upset!

Two weeks later, I came up with an excuse not to attend the Thursday youth meeting, and this continued the next week, and the next. That's when I realized that while I'd started attending for the right reasons, my later attendance was for the wrong reasons. Without meaning to, I made Mike my idol. It was all about Mike. I'm going back on a regular basis again, and this time for the right reasons." —Shannon Aldridge, 16

"Oh God, I Think Though Hast Outdone Thyself!"

—Edna St. Vincent Millay

As we saw with Shannon, something (or someone) can become an idol even without our knowing it—as was also true for 16-year-old Nick Hallenbeck, whose "idol" wasn't a person but, rather, nature.

> *I really like to surf. Not so long ago, that's all I wanted to do. When I was riding the waves, I was in heaven! When I wasn't surfing, I was thinking about it, dreaming about it, waxing my board, making plans in my head. It was an all-consuming passion. Go to church or go to the beach? No-brainer decision there! Surfing was way more important to me than it should have been. I do go to church now. I don't surf any less, but God doesn't take second to my surfing.* —Nick Hallenbeck, 16

Since the beginning of time people have idolized the forces of nature, even making up various gods to explain what they thought of nature's blessings. We gaze in awe at the majestic mountains, stare in wonderment at the seemingly endless ocean, speculate the height of a stately redwood tree, gawk at the edge of the Grand Canyon because we can hardly believe what our eyes are seeing. Still, nature is not a god. It does not bestow blessings. Yes, we look at God's creative genius in the variety of animals and realize in astonishment that all creation works together to sustain life. Still, it works together because of God. We touch a beautiful flower and are reminded of the words of Jesus who said, "Not even Solomon in all his splendor was dressed like one of these" (Matt. 6:29). Still, the beauty and splendor of a flower is painted by the hand of God.

No doubt about it, creation is more than awesome, and God wants His children to live within and amongst it! But not even the beauty of nature is to supersede our worship of God. The danger comes when we stargaze into nature and lose sight of the one true living God who created it. Perhaps you've heard someone say, "I don't go to church because I can look around and appreciate God in all I see." Yes, God wanted us to look at creation and realize its splendor. But we must know it is not for worship; it could not have come into existence without a genius of colossal proportions orchestrating its formation. That genius is God the Creator—and worthy of our worship!

Do You Have Idols?

Has anything come between you and God? What would you list that would qualify in your life as "idols"—things that overshadow your love for God as being at the core of your life? If so, have a talk with God about helping you restore Him to His rightful place in your life.

There's a story about a man named Thorwaldsen who carved a beautiful statue of Christ. The statue represented Jesus as having his hands outstretched and his head bowed. Someone who saw the statue complained, "I cannot see his face." The sculptor replied, "If you would see the face of Christ, you must get on your knees."

QUESTIONS FOR REFLECTION

- In what ways does God's second commandment apply to your life today?

- In what ways are the first and second commandments different?

- As in all the commandments, God guards something that is of great importance to our welfare. Why and how is the 2nd commandment important to your welfare?

- *"Teach me to do your will, for you are my God"* [Psalm 143:10a]? What does this Scripture mean to you?

- God wants to be first in our minds, hearts and in our lives. Why does God demand such "total" allegiance?

- We touch a beautiful flower and remember that Jesus said, *"Not even Solomon in all his splendor was dressed like one of these"* [Matthew 6:29]. When was the last time you looked around and felt as did Jesus? To what where you referring—a flower, a beauty of a certain person, a newborn kitten, or what?

- In what way would the world be different than it is now if everyone upheld God's second commandment?

5

THE THIRD COMMANDMENT

You shall not take [misuse] the name of the Lord Your God in Vain, for the Lord will not hold anyone guiltless who takes His name in vain.

Exod. 20:7

In each Commandment God guards something that is of the greatest importance to our welfare. In the previous chapter you learned how God commanded in His second law that we not worship or serve an idol of any kind. He is to be our One and only. By asking that we place our love for Him above all else, God is safeguarding our chance to truly know Him.

In this study of the third Commandment, we learn that God safeguards yet another avenue for our knowing and loving Him: When we say or hear His name, immediately our hearts should joyously identify Him as our Creator, our benevolent Heavenly Father, our Redeemer and Savior. Should we slander or diminish God's name, then our own disrespect will grow, and we may very well lose sight of all that God is to us. Therefore, we are not to dishonor His name in any way—and, we might conclude, we're to ask others to do likewise. We are to uphold His name as sacred and holy—as we profess when we say the Lord's Prayer: "Our Father, which art in heaven, hallowed be Thy name." The third Commandment, then, demands that we not misuse God's name, either by swearing, slandering, bearing false witness or deception. This Commandment has other implications as well: We should so love our Heavenly Father so that we call upon Him in times of need and, because we love Him, we should worship Him with praise and thanksgiving.

As always, our Father lets us know there are rewards for honoring this Commandment, and, likewise, consequences when we do not. In this case, the consequence is a part of the Commandment itself: "The Lord will not hold anyone guiltless who takes His name in vain." Upholding the third Commandment shows that we revere, love and trust God, and love each other as God loves each of us.

GOD'S THIRD COMMANDMENT IS STILL RELEVANT TODAY

Even some of the most revered among us use profanity as common language, and, in some places, young people aren't considered cool by their peers if they can't spew off cusswords as naturally as they might a smile. It's a time of not really knowing who is telling the truth. What does the third Commandment mean for you, living in a time of easy cheating, white lies and outright deception at seemingly every turn?

Why Is It So Important to God That We Keep His Name Holy?

Nothing could be more important for our welfare than God's name: "He makes the sun to rise . . . and sends the rain" (Matt. 5:45). Therefore, we must keep any and all the titles for which we address God as sacred, including Father, Creator, Jehovah, Redeemer, Jesus or Savior. All show His omnipotence. "God" means "source of all good"; "Jehovah" means "I am that I am." "Jesus," "Savior," "Almighty" and "Christ" mean "the anointed one" or "Messiah."

The name God stands for "His being"—which reveals Him to us. God allows us to know His name because He wants us to have a personal relationship with Him. We are to come to Him daily in prayer. We are to ask Him into our lives so that He will walk with us every day of our lives. He is a promise-making God, one who offers a generation-to-generation blessing, sealed by the gift of redemption. If we want the blessings that follow, we must never misuse His name. And why would we want to? He is our everything.

- God is the giver of life: "The Lord God breathed into his nostrils the breath of life, and the man became a living being" (Gen. 2:7).
- God is the granter of mercy: "Give thanks to the Lord, for He is good; His love endures forever" (Ps. 106:1).
- God is the source of soul-fulfillment: "Let them give thanks to the Lord for His unfailing love and His wonderful deeds for men! For He satisfies the thirsty and fills the hungry soul with good things" (Ps. 107:9).
- God is the wellspring of comfort: "He heals the brokenhearted" (Ps. 147:3); "Come to me, all you who are weary and burdened, and I will give you rest. Take My yoke upon you and learn from Me, for I am gentle and humble in heart, and you will find rest for your souls" (Matt. 11:28).
- God is the source of fellowship: "For where two or three come together in My name, there am I with them" (Matt. 18:20).
- God is the grantor of our prayers: "If you believe, you will receive whatever you ask for in prayer" (Matt. 21:22).
- God grants the desires within our hearts: "Ask and it will be given to you; seek, and you will find; knock, and the door will be opened to you" (Matt. 7:7).
- God is redeemer, giver of salvation and eternal life: "Praise the Lord, O my soul . . . who forgives all your sins and heals all your diseases, who redeems your life from the pit and crowns you with love and compassion, who satisfies your desires with good things" (Ps. 103:2–5).

God's blessings are mighty, and we should associate His name only with Holiness: "Praise the Lord, O my soul; all my inmost being, praise His holy name" (Ps. 103:1). By holding all that He stands for sacred and revered, we hold onto our opportunity to know Him as our Lord and Savior. We must never take His name in vain.

Here are three ways we show God that we revere, love and trust Him so as not to transgress against His third Commandment.

Three Ways We Keep God's Name Holy

1. We show respect for God's name. To use God's name without respect is one way we misuse His name. Even using God's name when not calling upon Him in reverence, such as in "Oh God, that test was brutal!" is showing disrespect for God.

    To me, respecting God's name shows up in the way we turn to God in times of need. Sometimes I need God for little things—like asking for help to get through some issue or problem, such as a semester final. And sometimes it's to help me through something big—like my grandfather's death. Two years ago, my grandfather passed away, and I felt so totally sad on some days, even mad. I just loved my grandpa so much; I'd lost a truly best friend. Gramps lived with us for the last few years of his life, and I got to know him and appreciate how much he loved me and supported me in my life. Sometimes I'd come home late from a game and there on my dresser would be a note congratulating me on our team's win or a positive message if we'd lost. He was just full of love and belief in me. I miss that more than I can put into words. Sometimes I still cry. I need God in these times. I know that God hears my prayers. I would encourage anyone NOT to use God's name in vain. I'd say that if you don't love God, if you don't know God. — Jimmy Van Norman, 20

2. We do not use profanity. Swearing is another way we break God's third Commandment. "Bless and do not curse," we are told in Romans 12:14. Do you swear? The Bible has much to say on this: "But I tell you, do not swear at all: either by heaven, for it is God's throne, or by the Earth, for it is His

footstool; or by Jerusalem, for it is the city of the great King. And do not swear by your head, for you cannot make even one hair white or black. Simply let your 'Yes' be 'Yes' and your 'No,' 'No'; anything beyond this comes from the evil one" (Matt. 5:34–37). Have you thought about why people curse God or swear?

Sometimes people swear because it's seen as "cool." I used to swear a lot when hanging around certain friends. At the time I considered it a "guy thing." But then I went to church camp and met some cool guys—and none of them swore. I decided that it wasn't so much a "guy thing" as it was just a bad habit my friends had. I don't swear anymore, because I think it's disrespectful to everyone, God included. —Weston Feldman, 16

Do you swear? If so, ask God to help you love Him more so that you stop disrespecting Him in this way. Cursing surely displeases our Lord: "Anyone who does these things is detestable to the Lord" (Deut. 18:12). We should make a conscious decision not to swear. We do this not only because God asks it of us, but because we have a responsibility to those around us: It can cause those around us to lose faith in God's Word.

While profanity has become so commonplace in today's times, something we take for granted, it is still a sin against our Heavenly Father. Can you think of any way in which we use God's name that is acceptable? For example, we carry coins in our pockets that are inscribed "In God We Trust." Is that okay with God?

Although the Word of God forbids swearing, it makes the exception for being sworn in as an officer of the law or as a witness. Christ himself testified under oath when the high priest appealed to Him (Matt. 26:63–64). In fact, one of the saddest moments in the Bible comes when Jesus was put under oath by Caiaphas the high priest who demanded: "I put you under oath by the living God; tell us if you are the Christ, the Son of God!" To this Jesus replied, "Yes, it is as you say . . . but, I say to all of you, in the future you will see the Son of Man sitting at the right hand of the Mighty

One, and coming on the clouds of heaven" (Matt. 26:64). This response simply exasperated the priest, who the Bible says, "tore at his clothing" and pronounced all as "blasphemy." You probably know the rest of the story (and if not, be sure to read the book of Matthew); all leads directly to the court saying, "He [Jesus] is worthy of death" (Matt. 26:66).

Once I told a friend something and she said, "Do you swear on a stack of Bibles?" When we want the ultimate truth, we refer to God as the ultimate 'you'd-better-or-else' proof to make sure we're getting it. —Lannie Glick, 13

3. We do not pervert God's Word. Perverting God's Word is another way we misuse His name. To "pervert" means to misrepresent. Throughout the Bible, God has much to say about this, especially in the book of Leviticus (19:11–18 NKJV): "You shall not steal, nor deal falsely, nor lie to one another. And you shall not swear by My name falsely, nor shall you profane the name of your God; I am the Lord. You shall not cheat your neighbor nor rob him. You shall not curse the deaf, nor put a stumbling block before the blind; I am the Lord. You shall do no injustice in judgment. You shall not be partial to the poor, nor honor the person of the mighty. In righteousness you shall judge your neighbor. You shall not go about as a talebearer among your people; . . . I am the Lord. You shall not hate your brother in your heart. You shall not take vengeance, nor bear any grudge against the children of your people, but you shall love your neighbor as yourself: I am the Lord."

How do we "pervert" God's Word? We misrepresent God when we "deceive by His name" or are hypocritical. People often do not recognize their own hypocrisy; they don't see how they are saying one thing and living another. For example, if we say we are Christians, but fail to abide by God's Commandments, then we are perverting the Word of God. "These people honor Me with their lips; but their hearts are far from Me" (Matt. 15:8). The following young people put this in context.

Some kids just go to my school because it has a reputation for having good teachers and because the classes are small and lots of kids get into college as a result. But that doesn't mean everyone who enrolls is necessarily a Christian. For some, while at the school they try to convince others they are a Christian, but when outside of school, don't act in Christian ways at all. — Bruce Walkins, 17

The way I see this hypocrisy playing out is that sometimes when I bow my head to pray in the cafeteria, some dude will come up and whap me on the head while I'm praying. Obviously, that's an intentional way of saying, "Oh look, a Jesus Freak." I'm somehow supposed to feel bad about asking God to bless my food, but when my grandmother died, this same kid said, "Sorry to hear about your grandma. My prayers are with you." I thought, "If your prayers are with me because I lost my grandma, then let your prayers be with me as I ask God to bless the food I eat." God is for all times so we should all see Him for all times. —Buddy Moreno, 14

Keeping God's Name Holy

Using God's name in disrespectful ways can stop your Christian growth. That's more reason to be vigilant, to watch your thoughts and words so they do honor God.

QUESTIONS FOR REFLECTION

- In what ways does God's third Commandment apply to your life today? In what ways is it still relevant?

- In what ways do you uphold the third Commandment?

- Why is it so important to God that you keep His name holy?

- Bearing false witness is another way we misuse God's name. Give an example of a time when you did this. Did you consider your action a sin against God?

- God wants us to keep any and all the titles for which we address God as sacred, be it Father, Creator, Jehovah, Redeemer, Jesus, Savior, Almighty or Christ. How do you feel when you hear any of these names taken in vain? What do you do about it?

- We carry coins in our pockets that are inscribed, "In God We Trust." Why do you think we put "In God We Trust"? Why not, "Have a nice day" or "spend wisely" or some other positive saying?

- Although the Word of God forbids swearing, it makes the exception for being sworn in as an officer of the law or as a witness. Why is this so?

- In what ways would the world be different if everyone upheld God's third Commandment?

STARVING CHILD

Oh, most gracious and loving God,
I sometimes wonder how You speak to us,
And how You get through to Your free-willed children.

I ask: Are You in the rib cage of a starving child,
... or the scream of an ambulance in the night,
... or the piercing sound of a hostile bullet?

Are You calling out in the shattering of an explosion,
... or when an angry knife stops a pulse,
... or a cruel word pierces a fragile heart?

Oh, most gracious and comforting God,
Are You saddened when Your children go astray,
... when a drunken parent hits a child,
... when a best friend dies of leukemia?

Do You grieve when Your children mess up their lives,
... too busy to come to You in prayer
... too full of ourselves to be grateful?

Oh, most gracious and forgiving God,
Thank You for loving and forgiving us
... when we think we can mend our own hearts
... and work our own miracles.

Oh, most gracious and redeeming God,
Teach us to make our will Your own,
... how to care for our brothers and sisters
... and to tend to our own souls.

Oh, most gracious Father and Creator,
Thank You for the evidence of Your abundant love,
... in the rising of the sun

. . . in the budding of a flower, and
. . . in the reassuring smile of a friend.

Every day You are right here beside us, and I know it.
Promising a new day and a fresh beginning.
Thank You most gracious and loving God.

—Kimberly Holcombe, 17

6

THE FOURTH COMMANDMENT

Remember the Sabbath day by keeping it holy . . .

Exod. 20:8

In the last chapter you learned it was of supreme importance to God that we not misuse His name; we are to guard it and keep it holy. We do this to preserve our own sense of God as omnipotent, and because upholding God's third Commandment shows our reverence, love and trust in our Heavenly Father. In this chapter, the study of God's fourth law, we learn that God once again asks us to "guard and keep holy" something. This time, it's the Sabbath, or Sunday.

Sabbath means rest. Saturday, the seventh day of the week, was the day of rest in the Old Testament. God gave the Sabbath to Israel for two purposes: First, as a day of rest: "There are six days when you may work, but the seventh day is a Sabbath of rest" (Lev. 23:3), and second, as a day of (public) worship, a time to hear and learn God's Word: "Six days you shall labor and do all your work, but the seventh day is a Sabbath to the Lord your God" (Exod. 20:9–10). The Sabbath, then, is a day to "tend to the needs of body and soul."

The Sabbath always has been a holy day for God. For those using the Roman calendar (most countries), it was on a Sunday that Christ arose from the dead (Easter Sunday). It was on a Sunday that the Holy Spirit was "poured out" and the church was born (Pentecost Sunday). But just as God lets us know that Sunday is the "Lord's Day," He also tells us it is our day: "For the Son of Man is Lord of the Sabbath" (Matt. 12:8). After letting us know that this day is a "gift" to us, we're instructed on how we're to use it: to rest and restore ourselves; and to worship and spend time (fellowship) with others.

As with all the other laws, we're to uphold this one. In Exodus 31:13 we hear, "You must observe My Sabbaths. This will be a sign between Me and you for the generations to come, so you may know that I am the Lord who makes you holy." And in Exodus 31:14 we learn that the misuse of it grieves God: "Observe the Sabbath, because it is holy to you. Anyone who desecrates it must be cut off from his people." Upholding the fourth Commandment shows that we revere, love and trust God, and love our "neighbors" as God loves us.

GOD'S FOURTH COMMANDMENT IS STILL RELEVANT TODAY

Again, in each Commandment God guards something that is of the greatest importance to our welfare. It's not so difficult to see why God's law was so needed over 4,000 years ago—a time of arduous and strenuous work and toil. After all, this was a time in which the demands of daily work were all-consuming, and worship was not just an automobile ride away. It was a time in which getting together with friends and relatives was perhaps a long journey, not just a matter of dialing them up, hopping on a plane or e-mailing the latest family photos. A day set aside for rest and worship was both a gift and a relief.

But that was then, and this is now. What possible reasons do we have to take a day of rest? Does the fourth Commandment still speak to us today? Can it help us learn to restore ourselves in ways that are meaningful to the self, to the soul and to the "neighbors" with whom we are making this earthly journey?

Is it a Sin to Work on Sunday (and Is Homework Considered Work)?

God expects us NOT to work on Sunday: "Six days you shall labor and do all your work, but the seventh day is a Sabbath to the Lord your God" (Exod. 20:9–10). Now that we're certain it is a sin to "labor" on Sunday, the question is, what does God mean by "work"? Are doing your homework, cleaning your room, doing chores or helping a friend fix up his new apartment considered "work"? What about shopping for groceries, going to your part-time job or taking a babysitting job down the street?

How does God define "work"? We know in some cases that God healed the sick on Sunday, or, as we learn in Matthew 12:8, Jesus went through the grain fields on the Sabbath when his disciples were hungry. And in Matthew 12:10–12, we learn that when he saw a man with a shriveled hand and healed him, Jesus was himself asked, *"Is it lawful to heal on the Sabbath?"* To this He replied, *"If any of you has a sheep and it falls into a pit on the Sabbath, will you not take hold of it and lift it out? How much more valuable is a man than a sheep! Therefore, it is lawful to do good on the Sabbath."* Does this mean, then, that it is okay to work on the Sabbath under "special circumstances"—for example, when a plumber or doctor responds to an emergency call for his or her services? Is it wrong for a retail business or a restaurant to open their door for business on Sunday, or if working on Sunday implies the business owner is not a "practicing Christian"?

SUNDAY: A DAY TO REST AND RESTORE OURSELVES

The Commandments are the basis for moral and spiritual conduct, as well as the foundation of peace and prosperity for the individual. Setting aside Sunday as a day to rest and sing praises to God was a practice that started during the time of the apostles, as we can see in Acts 20:7 and 1 Corinthians 16:2, as well as Revelation 1:10. Although steeped in the history of biblical times, this Commandment has application for today's times. What could be more important in these uncertain times of fast-paced schedules filled with stress and duress than that we observe Sunday as a day to rest, relax and restore ourselves?

Sunday is a hallowed day. "The Lord blessed the Sabbath day and made it holy" (Exod. 20:11). Using it as it was intended brings many opportunities and blessings. Still, as you look around the "real world" and see so many people working away on Sundays, are you wondering if we've forgotten (or are denying) the fourth Commandment? Natalie Brown, sixteen, discovered the importance of using Sunday in the way God intended.

My life was once so crazy. There was always so much to get done all the time that I found myself always so tired. Sunday was just another busy day, even though I wasn't at school.

All week long I have to get up at 6:30 to get ready for school, and on Saturdays I must be at work by eight o'clock. Sunday was the only day I had to get the tons of homework done. My life was so hectic and tiring, my parents told me I could no longer work the Sunday shift and that I had to start attending church with them again.

So now on Sundays I get to sleep in. Then I get up and go to the eleven o'clock Sunday service with my family, and later in the day, I spend time with friends. This "re-ordering of priorities" has been good. I'm a real fan of God's fourth Commandment! —Natalie Brown, 16

SUNDAY: A DAY FOR PUBLIC WORSHIP

Upholding God's fourth Commandment means that we also observe Sunday as a day of worship. While we should glorify the Lord every day of the week—by coming to Him daily in prayer and studying His Word in daily devotions—God asks that we use Sundays specifically to come together for public worship. Why? Why can't we just devote time on Sunday to reading and studying God's Word? Can't watching a televised church service, suffice? Why is God so specific about "public" worship?

Church: A Spiritual Family

The answer is that God wants us to view the church as a "spiritual family." Just as in your own family, each person is "looked out for" in a church family. First, membership in a church gives you identity. Attending church means we are likely to come to know each other. This is what God wants, even expects of us. God tells us that He considers it the duty of a Christian to pray for the church as a "holy institution," and to pray for the spiritual well-being of all its members, including its pastors, teachers and others who further the Word of God on behalf of the church. We are expected to support the church and its goals—such as provide Sunday school to the young and bring the Word of God to every member who belongs to our congregation. We are to carry the Word of God to other members of the congregation who cannot be in attendance, either because they are ill, infirmed, incarcerated or whatever else keeps them from hearing the Word of God. And yes, maybe just because they've become complacent, "too busy" or lost hope.

We are to tend even to those members who are in attendance. Some need us for encouragement to stay attached to the church while in the throes of their own challenging times. Others need someone to help lift a burden from their shoulders. Whether it is through our charitable contribution or by praying for them, we are to support the members of our spiritual family in their Christian walk—both in spirit and in person.

Does this mean that if we don't belong to a church that we are relieved of helping others to love and trust in God? No. Because we recognize God as the source and center of life, we gather in His name to help and support each other in our spiritual lives. This is the importance of membership in a group that shares your faith, and of coming together for public worship. Some people believe they needn't go to church, temple or a holy place to pay tribute to God. They believe that God hears them no matter where they are, and that is good enough. This interpretation misses the point of why God asks us to come together publicly. Publicly we come to the "throne of grace" in petition, in praise, in confession and intercession. "Let us go to the house of the Lord" (Ps. 122:1). Side-by-side with others, shoulder-to-shoulder, we acknowledge that He is worthy of our praises sung together: "There is no one holy like the Lord, there is no one besides You. There is no rock like our God" (1 Sam. 2:2).

We're to Attend Church Gladly and, Yes, Stay Awake While There

God delights in seeing us come together in His name. And by the way, He expects us to come willingly, even "gladly." And yes, once there, He expects us to stay awake, unlike Eutychus, who when Paul was giving a sermon, nodded off to sleep and fell out of the window, hitting his head so hard they thought the sleepy-head had killed himself! *Seated in a window was a young man named Eutychus, who was sinking into a deep sleep as Paul talked on and on. When he was sound asleep, he fell to the ground from the third story and was picked up dead* (Acts 20:9). (Later they discovered he hadn't died—but it's doubtful Eutychus ever fell asleep during a sermon again!)

God is pleased when He sees His people worship Him. Where God's Word is being preached, then good and truth and light are being shared. Reading the Scriptures and studying God's Word help us to better know God. We misuse Sunday when we make light of the preaching of God's Word or stay away from church services for a poor excuse, or for no reason at all.

How about you? Do your Sunday plans include worshiping your Heavenly Father?

SUNDAY: A DAY FOR FELLOWSHIP

We observe Sunday as a day of fellowship with others. God's fourth law asks that in addition to making Sunday a day away from work and a time of public worship, we use it as a time to gather together. God wants us to use Sunday as a time to honor Him by celebrating the ties that hold our families and our communities together. He's even promised to "be there" among us: "For where two or three come together in My name, there am I with them" (Matt. 18:20).

In addition to benefiting from setting aside a specific day for rest, recuperation, and social and celebratory time with family and friends, we're to make time to bring the Word of God—which can sometimes take the form of simply bringing our own happy heart and godly spirit—to someone who needs it. This would include making time on Sundays for visiting the sick, shut-ins and others who need spiritual nourishment. We are to use this day to visit those whose spirits need fresh air, such as people in hospitals or the elderly in nursing homes. "Religion that God our Father accepts as pure and faultless is this: to look after orphans and widows in their distress, and to keep oneself from being polluted by the world" (James 1:27).

How do you honor God in this way? Who in your community can benefit from your own happy heart, from all that you must share?

Being needed is such a positive thing, isn't it? Eleven-year-old Mary Gellens does this by taking her dog to the local children's cancer ward for the kids to pet and play with every other Sunday. Doing this helps take the children's minds off the painful chemotherapy treatments. There are so many ways that you are needed, too. Find something you can share, and then do it! It is sure to change your life, or at the least, have a positive effect on the person you're helping, something that 16-year-old Sara Tobias discovered.

I'm dating a guy from school who is a Christian. One of the ways he and I spend time together is by my going with him and his family to church on Sunday mornings. After that we go to his house for a big Sunday meal. It's their family ritual—a big meal where family and friends come together.

I love time at their house because the meal is never rushed, and everyone shares things going on in their lives. My family isn't like this at all. I live with my mom; my dad is remarried and lives in another state. I don't have any brothers or sisters.

No one goes to church. My mother doesn't, so I didn't until I started dating my boyfriend.

I'm hoping my mom will start going to church. She never went to church as a child, so it's not something that was a part of her life. But I can see her warming up to the idea because when I get back on Sunday afternoons, she is home and we talk about things. Before, she'd say, "Hi! Did you have fun?" and I'd say, "Yes, thanks for asking," and head to my room. Now, because I really want her to go to church so she can hear God's Word and to be with others who can help her feel welcome, I make a point of talking with her about it. I think it's because I'm in a "good space" and that contributes to the both of us being in a "good space." I'm hoping all this will help her decide to join a church.

When I get married and have a family, I'm going to do Sundays the same way my boyfriend's family does. There's something very special about coming together with others, praying together and just enjoying each other's company. I like the loving and peaceful yet empowering energy it creates. Because of my boyfriend, I've learned about God, and to honor his Commandments. —Sara Tobias, 16

PRESERVING THE GIFT OF A DAY SET ASIDE

God wants us to not permit anything to rob us—and Him—of the blessings of the day of rest, worship and fellowship. "Let us consider how we may spur one another on toward love and good deeds. Let us not give up meeting together, as some are in the habit of doing" (Heb. 10:24–25). How do you keep Sunday as holy as God wants?

What are your plans to be in "fellowship"—to socialize with your friends, and to help and assist those who need spiritual renewal? Think about it and make a goal. Whether this is a phone call to a grandparent—a call in which you are leisurely listening to your grandmother or grandfather and aren't watching the clock. This is the purpose of the Sabbath. Honor it: This is how you say thank you to our Heavenly Father for giving us His gift of rest for the "body, mind and soul."

QUESTIONS FOR REFLECTION

- In what ways do you uphold God's fourth Commandment?

- In what ways do you use Sundays to restore yourself?

- Do you attend church? In what ways do you feel that being a member of a congregation adds to your being involved in the church "community" — such as food drives and attending youth camp?

- Why does God set Sunday apart? Why does He provide guidelines on what we can and cannot do on this day?

- List two of your favorite contemporary Christian bands you most enjoy.

- Is it a sin to work on Sunday? What about doing homework or cleaning your room — is that considered "work"? Is it okay to work at a job on Sunday, especially if it's "serving" others? Is it okay for a plumber or doctor to respond to an emergency call for their services?

- "For where two or three come together in My name, there am I with them" (Matt. 18:20). What does this Scripture mean to you?

- In what ways would the world be different if everyone upheld God's fourth Commandment?

THE CRUCIFIX AROUND MY NECK

I wear a crucifix around my neck,
All day, every day, wherever I go.
No, it's not a fashion statement, not an "in thing,"
Nor is it to persuade those who say it isn't so.

I wear a crucifix around my neck,
A symbol of my faith in Christ,
Who thought of me in dying moments,
A most incredible and precious sacrifice.

I wear a crucifix around my neck,
Because he loved me from the start.
He knew my strengths, my faults, my sins,
And gave his life for me—what heart.

I wear a crucifix around my neck,
Thanking him for everything I see.
I wear it in his memory, then and now,
Because he sacrificed his life for me.

I wear a crucifix around my neck,
For his glory, I love him, I truly do.
I am not ashamed to say or show it,
In him I've found a life that's real and true.

I wear his crucifix around my neck,
It's him I choose eternally.
I am not afraid of death—nor life—because
I've secured my place in eternity.

—Laura Campanelli, 20

7

THE FIFTH COMMANDMENT

"Honor your father and your mother so that you may live long in the land the Lord your God is giving you."

Exod. 20:12

In the previous chapter, you learned that God set Sunday apart from the other days of the week, declaring it a holy day and instructing that it be used as a day to rest, worship publicly and encourage fellowship. In this study of God's fifth Commandment, God moves on from His teaching us how to focus our love and lives around Him and begins to instruct us on how to express our love to others. As you recall from the introduction, Jesus divided his laws into two parts—love for God and love for man. The first four Commandments teach love for God, and the last six teach love for our neighbor.

The fifth Commandment has been called the "centerpiece of the Commandments" because it involves both our relationship to God and to our fellow man. Our love for others flows out of our love for God. This Commandment requests that we honor and respect our parents, as well as those in other positions of authority: "Rise in the presence of the aged, show respect for the elderly" (Lev. 19:32). As you can see by the last part of the Commandment, God shares one of the consequences for upholding His law, "so that you may live long in the land the Lord your God is giving you." Upholding the fifth Commandment shows that we revere, love and trust God, and love our "neighbors" as God loves us.

59

In this Commandment, the words "mother and father" are symbolic. While the phrase "mother and father" most definitely refer to your own parents, God uses these words to represent "family" in broader terms (as you'll see in the coming pages). The Commandment is broad in scope in other areas as well, demonstrating that a Christian is to think of himself or herself as a member of three families—home, state and church. God has much to say about the importance of all three.

As you already know, in each Commandment God guards something that is of the greatest importance to our welfare. Like the others, this important fifth Commandment provides direction as to what we should and should not do, this time as it relates to God's definition of "family" in the context of our responsibilities to home, state and church. It's important to have guidelines for how we are to behave anytime people come together in a group, whether at home among family members, as part of a community or when communing with our "brothers and sisters" in the world.

GOD'S FIFTH COMMANDMENT IS STILL RELEVANT TODAY

It's not a stretch to understand how this Commandment was important in days of old. In a time when people had to cope with the elements, forage for food and build their own shelter, they needed to look out for others—especially those who were dependent, such as the young, the ill and the aging. It's understandable that when the population was expanding, specified boundaries for governing daily life, including its villages and towns, became necessary, but what about today?

Can the fifth Commandment help us to sort out our world as we know it today? Does it still provide direction for dealing with family, church and state?

WHO IS "YOUR FATHER" AND "YOUR MOTHER"?

Obviously, a mother and father—be they biological, adopted or surrogate parents—are "family." But this Commandment has meaning even beyond the two, three or four adults we call "Mom" and "Dad." Consider how Jesus referred to the wider sense of family. When Jesus was speaking to the multitudes someone said to him, "Your mother and brothers are standing outside, wanting to speak to you." Jesus replied, "Who is my mother, and who are my brothers?" Pointing to his disciples, he said, "Here are my mother and my brothers. For whoever does the will of my Father in heaven is my brother and sister and mother" (Matt. 12:47–50).

In 1 Timothy 5:1–3, we learn that "family" has an even larger membership: "Do not rebuke an older man harshly but exhort him as if he were your father. Treat younger men as brothers, older women as mothers, and younger women as sisters, with absolute purity. Give proper recognition to those widows who are really in need." Scripture even explains a bit of our responsibility to "family" by saying, "But if a widow has children or grandchildren, these should learn to put their religion into practice by caring for their own family and so repaying their parents and grandparents, for this is pleasing to God. If any woman who is a believer has widows in her family, she should help them and not let the church be burdened with them, so that the church can help those widows who are really in need" (1 Tim. 5:4, 16).

Regardless of their origin, parents are incredibly important to God—and He expects us to hold them in the highest regard. But He also asks a great deal of them, as well. For starters, God expects parents to be leaders in their homes. Let's see what this means.

Family Leadership: Who "Runs" the "Show" at Your House?

The fifth Commandment is not only for our own good, but for the sake of those with whom we share our lives. Imagine if there were no leadership in your home, or if everyone did his or her own thing regardless of how that affected the other members. This can result in divorce when one or both parents place their own desires above the needs and well-being of all family members. Even children can bring dissension in the family. Perhaps you've seen the effects yourself when one member of the family starts looking out only for his or her own well-being or special interests. This happened to 16-year-old Dana Hartford, who tells of her ordeal: *"When my older sister was 17, she decided no one should tell her what to do. To make her point, she was belligerent and uncooperative, not only to our parents but to me as well. She didn't care how it affected anyone else in the family. Our home was turned into a battlefield. We could no longer plan things because we couldn't count on her. It was like my sister was running the whole show. Everyone in the whole family was miserable because of her."*

As Dana learned, in order to create family harmony, each family member has responsibilities and common courtesies that must be followed so that there is order in the household. While the fifth Commandment assigns the leadership of children to the adults, it then gives children instructions on honoring and praying for their parents. All of this has bearing on the happiness of the "institution" of family.

The fifth Commandment's instructions for parents are to pray for their children; house, feed and clothe them; protect them from harm and danger; comfort them in sorrow; and watch over them in sickness. Their duties include nurturing their children, as well as guiding and instructing them in the Word of God. Such is the charge that God gives parents. What if parents do not do these things—are children given license to be angry with and disobey their parents? Not according to God, who says, "Cursed is the man who dishonors his father or his mother" (Deut. 27:16).

WHAT DOES GOD EXPECT OF YOU—YOUR PARENTS' CHILDREN?

God provides direction to you, the children, as well, regardless of how young or old you are. God asks that children honor, serve, obey, love and esteem their parents. In fact, children are even charged with protecting the "good name" of their parents. Regardless of what you personally think of your parents—whether you think they are "good" parents or not—God asks that children pray for their parents and for themselves. God calls for obedience when you feel your parents are wrong; God calls for respect even if you feel your parents do not deserve it; and God calls for loyalty even when your parents seem to be unreasonable. Does this mean that parents are always right or always do what is best? No. But God doesn't instruct us to obey only when we think they're right! He doesn't leave this judgment up to the kids—regardless of how old and wise we are! We are to honor, respect and obey our parents— and we are to do this because God says so. God asks kids—young and old alike—to bring their concerns about their parents to Him. After all, God is our Father, too—our Heavenly Father.

Why Life in the Family IS the "Real World"

God knows that what we learn by being a member of a family is vital to living among others in the "real world." Maybe that's why we humans have within our nature a desire to be with others. How many of your friends would rather stay alone in their rooms as opposed to being invited by others to spend time and fellowship with them? Every now and then we get a little tired of always being around others—but mostly we prefer the company of others rather than isolation.

The more time we spend with others, the better we understand the rules for getting along. This is a good thing. No one likes to be with selfish, self-centered, arrogant, "it's-all-about-me" kinds of people. This is another reason why learning to be a "member" of your family at home is a good thing. For example, in addition to learning how to share and look out for the comfort and well-being of others, one of the values your parents are trying to instill is to have a healthy respect for authority. Authority teaches self-control, patience and tolerance, among other things—all essential qualities to living life on your own and being with others. Having a mind-set for looking out for others and a heart generous enough to care about the comfort of others are the hallmarks of understanding that you're sharing your time here on Earth with others, and for a reason.

Being a member of a family teaches you all these things and more. Being a member of a family IS the real world. What you learn there is what you will carry into the world each day—starting with today. See the wellbeing of each family member as important as your own. Learning to be responsible in pulling your weight helps everyone enjoy and respect one another and strengthens your family bond.

> *It seems to me that my some-time friend, Raynelle, runs her family. She always seems to get her way, yet she's always complaining, always wanting something, and it's not like her family can afford it. She acts entitled, like she deserves everything. Raynelle is in four of my classes—so we see each other a lot, but I don't consider her a "good friend" because she only thinks of herself.* —Michelle McCabe, 15

Being a member of a family is in the best interest of everyone. By honoring their parents, children show that they love God and become a blessing to their parents.

WHAT DOES GOD SAY ABOUT THE RESPONSIBILITY OF YOUR PARENTS?

As you've figured out by now, God's laws are so perfectly thought out that they benefit everybody—which is why this Commandment is not a one-way street. Parents have obligations, too—in fact, far more than their children do!

Besides caring for their children's physical needs, parents are expected to live a life characterized by integrity, honesty, responsibility and faith in God. They are instructed to earn and be worthy of their children's love and obedience. Prayer and family devotions are a part of their responsibility. And they are to teach their children self-control. God goes so far as to ask parents to correct children when they are not being obedient, saying, "Do not withhold discipline from a child" (Prov. 23:13).

This does not give parents a license for being unfair. God lectures, "Fathers, do not exasperate your children; instead, bring them up in the training and instruction of the Lord" (Eph. 6:4). Most of all, God expects parents to teach their children about God and to demonstrate—through their own behavior—God's love, as we learn in Proverbs 22:6: "Train a child in the way he should go, and when he is old, he will not turn from it."

Five Ways to Honor Your Parents and God

1. **Love your parents.** The older you get, the more you want to take control of your life. That is as it should be. Still, listen to what your parents have to say. Allow them to shape your character—to help you always to see life from the eyes of your heart, and to learn about God's love so that you will want to be a person who walks with God. Maybe your parents do that already. Maybe they don't know how to do that; maybe they're still trying to come to terms with their own hurts and wounds from the past. Maybe their own lives are filled with chaos, and it spills over into your own, making for a difficult relationship between the two of you. If this is the case, ask for God's guidance in loving and honoring your parents. Have you ever asked God to lead you into a better relationship with your parents? God wants you to, and it's sure to give you insight on how to make your family life better.

   Do all you can to love your parents. Do all you can to create a happy home for all the members of your family. Don't expect your parents to be perfect just because they're older. Each day you get out of bed is the first day they've had the opportunity to be your parents on that day. It may be difficult to believe, but parents are learning as they go, too. Does this absolve them of the responsibility to be effective parents? No, but it can help you see them as being mere humans. Do all you can to create a relationship "for the long haul."

   Like others my age, I felt my parents were too strict, but it wasn't long after I left home that I could see the benefits of all

I had learned from them and realize how fully I loved them. Thankfully, my parents and I shared nearly five decades of mutual love and admiration. Other than my relationship with God, to be one of their children was the greatest gift I've ever been given. Such is the power of the bond we can form with our parents. I wish it for you and hope you will do your part to be a "happy" family.

While it can seem like parents are "behind the times," too strict or not "cool" enough be assured that your own future children will feel just as you do sometimes. That's just the way it works! God has a plan—and you're in it!

Vow to love and honor your parents. Ask God to grant you the peaceful and loving heart that makes you a joy and blessing to your parents.

2. **Obey the house rules—and look for the love behind them.** It's always difficult to color within the lines, but sometimes it's the only way to get a picture to turn out the way it's supposed to be! Likewise, when you follow the rules your parents have set, you are more likely to be safe and to feel like you are loved. You will see your own (good) character emerge.

    What if you feel the rules are too strict or out of line? Then try this: Think about each rule, and then write each one down. Next, write out what you feel is the reason for each of the rules. Then, draw a line, making two columns. In one column, list all the possible benefits for following the rules, and in the next column, list all the ways the rule protects you or serves you. Now study it. Do you still wish for some change? If so, have a talk with your parents and agree on ways you can do that. The bottom line is that parents enjoy it when their children learn and grow and change. Most all parents look forward to their children learning to "stand on their own two feet." Being able to make wise choices helps your parents see that you are not only growing up but growing wise. Often the trick to peaceful coexistence is talking things out.

3. **Learn to be a good communicator—and ask God to sit in on family discussions.** Because you are getting old enough to make decisions of your own, you may very well need to

talk with your parents about what the rules are and how to cocreate new ones. If you still need to work on discussion and negotiation skills, don't wait for your parents to learn and apply them. Get busy and do this for yourself. Start by being a good listener. Learn how to express yourself in ways that assure you will be listened to and taken seriously. Ask God to sit in on things. Learn to say, "Let's pray about this, and talk again"—which can make all the difference in his relationship with his parents.

4. **Be appreciative and practice saying, "thank you."** Think about the times when someone appreciated sincerely something you've done and told you so. Didn't that make you feel good about yourself? Didn't the fact that you'd been praised bond you to the person who expressed satisfaction? Quite often, parents don't get the praise and thanksgiving they deserve. Just because parents are "supposed" to care for you, don't neglect to show your gratitude. Make it your honor—as much as it is your obligation to God—to show gratitude for all your parents do for you. This can be simple, such as, "Dad/Mom, thank you for taking me to school this morning." Or "Thank you for being my dad (or mom)." Or "Thank you for cheering me on at my game yesterday. It helped me to feel more confident." An attitude of gratitude is pleasing to your parents. Moreover, it is pleasing to God.

5. **Look out for your siblings.** On my parents' fiftieth wedding anniversary, they gathered us kids together for a dinner. Immediately following the meal, they handed each of us a half sheet of paper upon which they had typed a "message" for us to always keep—words they wanted us to take to heart. It said, *"Please always love each other. Take care and look after each other. Raise God-loving children. If you do this, we will feel that we have been, in some way, good parents."* This was followed by the following Scripture: "If your brother sins against you, go and show him his fault, just between the two of you. If he listens to you, you have won your brother over. If he will not listen, take one or two others along so that 'every matter may be established by the testimony of two or three witnesses.'. . . I tell you, that if two of you on Earth agree about

anything you ask for, it will be done for you by My Father in heaven. . . . Then Peter came to Jesus and asked, 'Lord, how many times shall I forgive my brother when he sins against me? Up to seven times?' Jesus answered, 'I tell you, not seven times, but seventy-seven times'" (Matt. 18:15–16, 19, 21–22).

What we children learned was that of all the things our parents had done in their roles as parents, they considered that our loving each other, and caring for each other the way God intended, was the mark of their having succeeded as parents. If one of us were to step out of line, we were to go and convince that person to come back to the fold. "A healthy family always claims each other," they told us. "No matter what, and under all conditions, whether it be in times of celebration or chaos, love each other and take care of each other." That little slip of paper has remained so important to each of us children that we each still have it—for some of us, framed and on a wall. Amazing what God-guided love can do!

Most parents want their children to love, look after and always "be right" with their siblings. Do this because you love your parents. Do this because you want to grow in love for your brothers and sisters. Do this because you love God. It is because of His love that you are learning, day-by-day, the importance of loving all His children, everywhere.

THE "FAMILY" OF GOVERNMENT: WHAT DOES GOD SAY IS ITS DUTY TO ITS PEOPLE?

Did you think that the government was though up by us earthlings? Not so. Scripture is filled with God's mandates how the "state" must be organized and how it is to conduct itself in the "fair dealings" (treatment) of His people. God does not want us to look at government as being an impersonal entity. God wants us to see the government as an extension of our willingness to care about and for each other—to look after His children's well-being.

Who is the "state"? The state is the "larger family"—meaning all those who "live in the land." This may be a city, a town or the geographic boundaries of a state. According to God, the duty of a government is to govern in accordance with the laws of the land.

It's easy to see that, without this, there would be neither law nor order. God directs that government is to work for the people. Does God have something to say to our litigious society? You bet: "Settle matters quickly with your adversary who is taking you to court. Do it while you are still with him on the way, or he may hand you over to the judge, and the judge may hand you over to the officer, and you may be thrown into prison" (Matt. 5:25).

Ideally, it's up to the people to decide what form of government they wish to be under. The responsibility of the government should be that it faithfully works for the welfare of the people according to the laws it has set forth. It is the duty of this government to be honest and just, and to protect those who follow its laws, as well as to punish those who do not. Does God demand that the rulers be just, impartial and trustworthy? You bet. He demands it: "He does not bear the sword for nothing. He is God's servant" (Rom. 13:4). If you're thinking that God expects us to pray for our leaders and for our government, you would be correct.

To the citizen God says, "Everyone must submit himself to the governing authorities" (Rom. 13:1). What if the leader (hence the government) is corrupt? Are you willing to pray for oppressive leaders? Above all, God expects us to obey Him over all others, saying, "Give to Caesar what is Caesar's, and to God what is God's" (Matt. 22:21). If you take this one step further, you will see that incorporated into this Commandment is a promise to nations, as well. While the promise in this Commandment was especially given to Israel, it is also a promise to all nations who uphold its meaning. A nation that honors fathers and mothers because it fears and loves God—because it "walks righteously"—will be strong morally and physically. The individual shares in the safety and blessings that doing so brings.

WHAT DOES THE FIFTH COMMANDMENT SAY ABOUT YOUR OBLIGATION TO THE GOVERNMENT?

What does it mean to honor the state, and in what ways can you personally do your part? As a young adult, there are many ways you can make a difference in honoring the "state." Practically speaking, honoring the state means the obvious, like not breaking the laws against shoplifting, stealing and killing. But it also means to obey the laws of the land, such as no speeding or running stop signs. It means paying taxes that we owe and not cheating. It means not throwing trash out the windows of your car, thereby marring the countryside. It means praying for our leaders that they would have "the mind of Christ" as they make decisions in governing our country. It means doing your part to support the country so that we can function harmoniously as a "family." And more.

Four Ways You Can Honor the "Family" of Government

1. **Value freedom, and don't take it for granted.**

    I'm far more aware of how lucky I am to live in a country that values freedom and thank God every day for the freedoms I enjoy. When I sing the National Anthem, I think about how God has blessed our country, and pledging allegiance is more of a prayer. Since my awareness has been heightened, I'm a better citizen. I'm more courteous to others, I'm more polite, and I speak up about the importance of freedom and everything related to it. I pray for our soldiers who are risking their God-given lives so that we can maintain the freedoms we enjoy. And I have much to say about governments who do not create freedoms for their people. I have become, I've discovered, an activist. —Jonathan Bridges, 14

2. **Obey the laws.**

    I just got my driver's license. Last week I changed lanes even though I could tell it would be a close call, and nearly hit another car. Speed limits, traffic lights and stop signs are put there for our safety, and when I disregard them, I put others in danger. That's not what I want to do. I count obeying the traffic laws as one way to uphold God's fifth Commandment.
    —Bethany Oglethorpe, 16

3.   Vote for those who stand for the values of justice, fairness and honesty.

*I no longer vote for someone simply because that person is my friend or more popular than someone else who may be running for office. I take my voting power seriously and really try to think who the best person for the job will be. I think it's exactly what this mandate from God is about. —*Jennifer Hanson, 17

4.   Pray for the leaders of your country.

*My favorite book is Lord of the Flies. A group of little boys survive a plane crash and are marooned on an island. Without realizing what they are doing, the first thing they do is to set up their own government with rules and responsibilities for everybody. But because there is no one to enforce adherence, the government begins to break down and chaos breaks loose—at its worst, they begin killing each other. Those little boys represent who we are without God, and the anarchy shows what we'd be like without government. God in His love and wisdom gave us government. —*Dan Deerborne, 20

WHAT DOES GOD SAY ABOUT THE OBLIGATION OF THE CHURCH TO YOU— AND YOU TO THE CHURCH?

Because we recognize God as the source and center of life, we gather in His name. There are some who believe they needn't go to church, a temple or holy place to pay tribute to God. Some people believe God hears them no matter where they are, and so that is good enough—wherever they are, they are already with God. This is not how God sees it. God asks that we use Sundays specifically to come together for public worship. This can encourage and support others in their Christian walk. When we lift our voices in praise to Him, side by side with others, we encourage others to know God more fully. This is the power of belonging to a church—and how doing so serves your Christian walk. You must give back.

The church is a spiritual family. As a "church" family, we look out for the spiritual "health" of each other. It is the duty of a Christian to pray for the church, along with its pastors, teachers and other workers. We are charged with knowing the functions of our church, and, moreover, we are expected to support the church and its goals—such as providing Sunday school and bringing the Word of God to those who cannot attend but would like to—such as the ill. We are each to do this to the best of our ability, and in accordance to the gifts and talents God has individually bestowed.

FOUR WAY YOU CAN HONOR THE "FAMILY" OF CHURCH

1. **Go to church.**

    If I stopped feeding my cat, she would die. And if I stopped going to church, I could die spiritually. I need spiritual food as well as what's in the refrigerator at home. —Gretchen Ashmore, 13

2. **Tithe.**

    I tithe not only because God expects me to, but because our sharing what we have with others is a part of God's plan to continue spreading the Word of God. God expects us to give money directly to the church so that it can fulfill its goals and obligations to any outreach ministries it has. —Christina Salazar, 16

3. **Accept God into your life.**

    Last year was the first time I'd ever gone to church. A friend invited me to go with him, and several weeks later, I accepted Christ into my life. To say I've never been the same would be an understatement to say the least! My life was boring, and, I'd have to say, kind of meaningless. But now, I'm on fire! I have purpose. I have direction. I have energy. I love life. Now my church is like family to me. I go now because it is the "juice" I need to keep me going. To keep me healthy. To keep me mentally and morally strong. —Dwayne Carter, 17

4. **Pal around with other Christians.**

My church youth group is the center of my social life. I've found all my best friends there because we share the same values and goals—our faith in Jesus. We study, learn and pray together, but we also play together; some of my best memories have been going to camps, amusement parks and skiing with my youth group. Because we all share the same faith, I don't have to worry about being pressured to do wrong things, and I can count on my friends to make sure that I don't get off track either. I can't imagine life without my Christian friends.
—Doug Donovan, 15

Family: A Brand of Love Unparalleled to Any Other

It is within our families that real life is played out. With them we let our hair down, relax and feel free to express our deepest needs, greatest fears and infinite hopes. It is with them that we feel able to discuss our hurts, pains and wounds. It is with them that we express feelings of love. After all, these are the people with whom we have laughed and cried, cooked and shared meals, and played and fought daily over many years. It is with these people that we can be ourselves. They've seen us at our arrogant best and, most assuredly, at our worst and lowest moments. And still, they love us. Home is where we turn to when we need to fill up our tanks with the brand of love that family reserve only for each other. It is a love unparalleled to any other.

Yes, the bonds of family are important to our lives. The strength of character we gain there will be our passport to living successfully in the world. Asking God to walk with us and guide us as we learn to love and appreciate each person in our families will be the mortar for the rooms we build within our hearts so that we have space to love others. How are you doing learning these things? Take to heart the advice in Philippians 2:4, "Each of you should look not only to your own interests, but also to the interests of others."

Ask God to help you create this within the context of your family.

QUESTIONS FOR REFLECTION

- Why is the fifth Commandment is called the centerpiece of the Commandments?

- The 5th commandment requests that we honor and respect our parents and not provoke them to anger. What do you think is meant by "do not provoke them to anger"?

- According to God's 5th law, children are not to be angry with their parents, "*Cursed is the man who dishonors his father or his mother*" (Deut. 27:16). What is God's reasoning for making this demand?

- God considers "the state" as a part of the "larger family." In what ways do you think of the state as an extension of family?

- The duty of a government is to govern in accordance with the "laws of the land," but up to the people to decide what form of government they wish to be under. Do you think we each have an obligation *to each other* to vote, and, to be conscious about our vote?

- God says we each are to pray for our leaders and for our government. Do you think prayer could help us improve the conditions of the world?

- God says that it is the duty of a Christian to pray for the church, along with its pastors, teachers, and other workers. Do you pray for your church in this way?

- God tells us that "public" worship is important because it through fellowship that we encourage and support each other in learning God's Word. In what ways do you worship "publicly"?

THE SIXTH COMMANDMENT

Thou Shalt Not Murder.

Exod. 20:12

In the previous chapter you learned that God instructed us to honor our fathers and mothers so our days are "long in the land." The sixth Commandment is about living long as well, but this time as it relates to the preservation of life. Because human life has eternal value to God, He created a law to protect human life against willful destruction.

This "value-of-life" Commandment has implications beyond taking the life of another. We're NOT to take the life of a fellow human being, but the Commandment protects beyond the number of days in which we're given to breathe. This sixth Commandment also declares that we are to care about others—and to the degree that we do them no bodily harm, nor cause them any suffering. We are told to help and befriend each other in every need. "Greater love has no one than this, that he lay down his life for his friends" (John 15:13).

Not only does God call for the protection of human life in His sixth law, but we are informed of the consequences if we disobey: "Whoever sheds the blood of man, by man shall his blood be shed. For in the image of God has God made man" (Gen. 9:6). Out of reverence, love and trust for God, and because we love others as God loves us, we abide by His Commandment.

75

GOD'S SIXTH COMMANDMENT IS RELEVANT TODAY

As with all the Commandments, God guards something that is of great importance to our well-being. It is not too difficult to understand that God is looking out for our interests when He commands that someone not murder us. God also tells us we're to not cause each other suffering—be it physical pain or emotional duress.

But what about in modern civilization?

How shall we apply the Commandment to crimes against race, creed, color and sexual differences, or as the multitude of school shootings suggest, against those who inflict pain or death upon others because they feel different, excluded or suffer from feelings of alienation? How does the Commandment sort out or justify the destruction of life, be it on death row, through suicide or an abortion? Does it offer any guidelines to keep drunk drivers off the road and drug dealers off the streets? Does the Commandment speak to the school bully tormenting the timid?

THE LOVE BEHIND THE LAW: TO GOD, EACH HUMAN LIFE HAS ETERNAL VALUE

The love behind God's sixth law is this: To God, all human life is sacred; each soul has eternal value. God's reasoning is straightforward. We each are God's creation: "So God created man in his own image, in the image of God. He created him; male and female He created them" (Gen. 1:27). God declares that each one of us belong to Him. A crime against another person's life is a crime against God. That alone should make us stop and think about inflicting death or emotional duress upon another. Consider what is at stake for God: When God looks upon His children, He sees the eternal possibilities. When you look at a good friend, perhaps your first "take" is "good friend; happy person; smart; makes me laugh; we like to spend time together," or something to that effect. While we see attributes or qualities, God sees a soul. In each of us, God sees the untold possibility for each of our lives to be with Him through-out eternity.

Under God, each of us shares the same birthright: We all have the opportunity for companionship with God. By living according to the Commandments set forth for our welfare, we each have a right to understand and take the walk that leads to being reunited with God. God wants each of His children to know eternal life.

God is serious about each life; no one must destroy or harm in any way that which is His.

Should we fear for ourselves if we transgress against God? Scripture provides ample evidence: "This day I call heaven and Earth as witnesses against you that I have set before you life and death, blessings and curses. Now choose life, so that you and your children may live and that you may love the Lord your God, listen to His voice, and hold fast to Him. For the Lord is your life and he will give you many years in the land he swore to give to your fathers, Abraham, Isaac and Jacob" (Deut. 30:19–20).

We, too, are to value life as sacred, knowing that each life begins as a gift from Him. We have an obligation to God to care for His children, so they may come to know God and share in the birthright of life everlasting.

DOES GOD MAKE A DISTINCTION BETWEEN MURDER AND KILLING?

Notice that the Commandment is more accurately translated as "You shall not murder" rather than "You shall not kill." If God had said the latter, then his explicit instructions to the Israelites as to how they were to annihilate the pagan tribes who were occupying the Promised Land would have been completely contradictory to his own instructions. What does this mean for us, living in a time in which our world is uncertain and volatile? Again, Scripture provides insight: ". . . a time for war and a time for peace" (Eccles. 3:8), and ". . . a time to kill and a time to heal" (Eccles. 3:3). We can conclude that soldiers protect the freedom and safety of citizens. Justified war, then, falls under the category of self-defense and is justified under God's laws. But this does not mean we are to regard war as something to be taken lightly: "Wisdom is better than weapons of war" (Eccles. 9:18), and "Make plans by seeking advice; if you wage war, obtain guidance" (Prov. 20:18).

Who, then, is a murderer? Is it only the person who kills intentionally, as in shooting someone to death? Or is it also applied to that person who, while driving recklessly or under the influence of drugs or alcohol, causes an accident in which someone loses his or her life? What if life is lost through assisted suicide or abortion?

God's Word: A Moral Compass
for Evaluating Moral Judgments

Luckily, we have God's Word to provide us with a moral compass for evaluating ways in which we inflict hurt, punish or take the life of another. What we learn is that God doesn't easily excuse us or let us off the hook. "If you suffer, it should not be as a murderer or thief or any other kind of criminal, or even as a meddler" (1 Pet. 4:15). God even has words for those of us whose "evildoings" remain locked in our heads. Says God, he who is angry with his brother also is guilty of murder. "You have heard that it was said to the people long ago, 'Do not murder, and anyone who murders will be subject to judgment.' But I tell you that anyone who is angry with his brother will be subject to judgment'" (Matt. 5:21–22). In the sight of God, hatred is the root of murder. It may never make us criminals, but it makes us sin against God.

God wants us to "clean house" on all thinking that is "hateful." God wants us to know that even neglecting to help others who need our support is, in fact, a selfish cruelty—and a sin against His Commandment. As future leaders of the world, you might even speculate as to the broader application of "murder." What might it mean for those who produce, sell and/or advertise cigarettes, liquor or other harmful substances? What about those who promote things, such as pornography, that destroy a person's spirit or desire to serve God? Isn't this, too, a sin against this Commandment? God goes so far as to say that even the motives for doing evil fall under the umbrella of murder: "Anyone who hates his brother is a murderer" (1 John 3:15). The consequences are dire: "You know that no murderer has eternal life in him" (1 John 3:15).

SUICIDE: IS IT A SIN?

To God our lives are precious: They are holy, sacred, blessed and consecrated. "God's temple is sacred, and you are that temple" (1 Cor. 3:17). But what if a person has an incurable disease or a terminal illness, making life seem unbearable? Might that be grounds for ending one's own suffering? God wants us to know that as the giver of life, He is the only one who has the right to end it. To take matters into our own hands can be viewed as our willful intention to usurp God's authority—to figuratively shake our finger at Him and say, "It's my life, and I'll do with it what I want." If we trust God with our lives, then we must also trust Him when it is our time to die.

If you've read *A Teen's Guide to Christian Living: Practical Answers to Tough Questions About God and Faith*, perhaps you remember a beautiful and heartfelt story called "Wounded Angel" by 18-year-old Genta Tyla Murry. In the story a young woman named Laura was suicidal and considered ending her life. Luckily, she got help for her depression. Still, the greatest insight for her understanding that she must choose life over suicide didn't come only at the hands of her excellent therapists. Reading the Bible one evening, she came to understand that she didn't have a right to take her life. "I eagerly expect and hope that I will in no way be ashamed but will have sufficient courage so that now as always Christ will be exalted in my body, whether by life or by death. For to me, to live is Christ and to die is gain. If I am to go on living in the body, this will mean fruitful labor for me. Yet what shall I choose? I do not know! I am torn between the two: I desire to depart and be with Christ, which is better by far; but it is more necessary for you that I remain in the body," she read in Philippians 1:20–24.

Laura said these words "ministered to my crying soul" and helped her realize that taking her life was against God's Word— and so she vowed to God that she never would. After all, if she loved God—and loved those around her as God loved her—then she must choose to live. Scripture had shown Laura that "to live" must be her goal.

We might ask ourselves, why does God allow us to suffer in the first place? God would have us know that for all our circumstances, uncomfortable and seemingly intolerable as they appear, He allows us to feel burdened at times, even for our will to be tested: "The Lord examines the righteous" (Ps. 11:5). In James 1:3–4 we learn that it can even be for our own good: "The testing of your faith develops perseverance. Perseverance must finish its work so that you may be mature and complete, not lacking anything." From these words we learn that, although our lives can be difficult, challenging times can make ups strong. Pain, heartache and sorrow cause us to mature, to deepen our faith and to grow closer to God.

Difficult times may cause us to question not only what we are doing, but why. Feeling sad and hopeless can move us closer to God, and so we turn our eyes heavenward. Certainly, we are assured that God will not give us more than we can bear. "No temptation has seized you except what is common to man. And God is faithful; He will not let you be tempted beyond what you can bear. But, when you are tempted, He will also provide a way out so that you can stand up under it" (1 Cor. 10:13).

These are heavy thoughts, aren't they? But knowing what God expects is comforting. Don't feel you have to shoulder life alone: No one expects anyone to have all the answers. Should you be facing overwhelming problems or feel sadness and despair, be sure to talk to an adult you trust. Have a talk with your youth pastor as well. And don't forget to take your burdens to God. God knows about despair; he knows of the shame we hide; he knows when we have heavy burdens. God affirms that nothing is too great to bring to Him. He will bring us peace. He will restore us. He will make us whole and new. When we have sinned and can hardly bear our shame, when we need renewal and a fresh start, know that God will grant it. "I will repay you for the years the locusts have eaten" (Joel 2:25).

We only need to ask. "If we confess our sins, he is faithful and just and will forgive us our sins and purify us from all unrighteousness" (1 John 1:9).

God Expects Us to Love Our Enemy: Is He Serious?

Loving ourselves is one thing, but what about our enemies? "Love your enemies, do good to those who hate you, bless those who curse you, pray for those who mistreat you" Christ commands in Luke 6:27–28. Is he serious? What does God mean when he says that we must love our enemies? He must know that in some cases, this is most difficult to do!

Rest assured, He means it. Jesus said, "If you love those who love you, what credit is that to you? Even 'sinners' love those who love them. And if you do good to those who are good to you, what credit is that to you? Even 'sinners' do that. But love your enemies, do good to them and lend to them without expecting to get anything back. Then your reward will be great, and you will be sons of the Most High. Be merciful, just as your Father is merciful" (Luke 6:32–36). What God means here is that we should not let the way someone treats us affect the way we treat him in return. This idea completely wipes out any thoughts we have of getting revenge or getting even. We cannot control how someone else acts; we only can control how we act.

God also says that we should pray for our enemies—that we should pray for good things to happen to them. And here's even more good news! Amazing things happen when we begin to pray for our enemies; it changes us! It's hard to nurse a grudge when you're praying for good things for someone. Why would Jesus suggest we bother loving our enemies? Because it is precisely the kind of love that mirrors the love God has for us. Nothing destroys our health, mars our countenance and robs our joy like hatred. It's the worst kind of illness. When we nurse anger, we are hurting ourselves. God would say for our own good to rise above it, act in a way we won't regret and move on.

Upholding God's Sixth Commandment

In the sixth Commandment, God asks us to not take the life of our fellow travelers. Because God models His love for us, we are likewise asked to model it for others. What does it mean to love our fellow human beings? It means that we are to help and befriend each other in their every need. We are to be our brother's keeper. How do we show God that we are grateful for our lives and respect the lives of His children everywhere? Here are some suggestions from teens and young adults.

1. **Don't be the cause of someone's death.**

    I try to be a good driver. I don't want to hurt or kill someone because of my carelessness. So that's one way I try to uphold this Commandment. I know that to God, life is sacred; it is to me, too. —Daniel Lathrop, 18

2. **Obey the laws designed to protect us.**

    I try to be very conscious about any way I may be a part of endangering someone else's life. I never drive "under the influence." I'd like to tell you that I never drink, but sometimes I do but I never drive at those times. And I make sure I never get into a car when the driver has had alcohol or used drugs. —Larry Rogers, 17

3. **Stop the "hate" in your home, school or community.**

    When I hear gossip, I make a point of saying something to get others to change the subject. If the gossip is malicious, I often say something like, "Gossip usually doesn't end well for anyone." When I do this, there'll usually be this moment of uncomfortable silence, but I'm okay with that. —MaryLynn Jones, 22

4. **Help others.**

    The other day I was riding to school with a friend. We pulled up to a stop sign, and there was a homeless person holding a "Will Work for Food" sign. My friend rolled down her window and gave him three dollars. When I remarked that her actions only encouraged him to beg for money, she replied, "He looked like he needed help, and I had some to give." Her comment helped me to examine my beliefs about helping others. My heart got bigger. —Marissa Gonzales, 16

5. **Care for your spirit.**

   I think it's important to take care of ourselves when we see ourselves getting overwhelmed or depressed. God does not want us to get so despondent or depressed that we consider ending the pain. When I feel at the end of my rope, I ask God or guidance and peace. —Jessie Marie Conley, 15

6. **Share the good news of Jesus.**

   There are so many people who need a loving, nonjudgmental response in their time of discouragement. I remember these words: "I was hungry and you gave me something to eat; I was thirsty and you gave me something to drink; I was a stranger and you invited me in; I needed clothes and you clothed me; I was sick and you looked after me; I was in prison, and you came to visit me. . . . Whatever you did for one of the least of these brothers of mine, you did for me" (Matt. 25:35–36, 40). This reminds me to help others, and I sometimes simply say to someone, "I will pray for you." —Ryan Phillips, 24

7. **Be a social activist.**

   Because business and politics are too often the instruments of injustice, it is the Christian's privilege and duty to take an active interest in the civic affairs of his community and country. Each of us must make sure that justice prevails, that security of life and home be guaranteed, and that each person has a right to earn a living. As God reminds us, "Anyone, then, who knows the good he ought to do and doesn't do it, sins" (James 4:17). —Leigh Kuiper, 28

Keeping God's Commandment

Perhaps when you started this chapter you thought, I never break this Commandment, because I've never murdered anyone! But now that you see the broader implications of the Commandment. If you feel there are some ways you've sinned against God, ask God for forgiveness. Then take positive steps to make amends. This may mean apologizing to someone you've wronged. It may mean changing habits—the way you act, the things you say. It may mean that you'll want to reach out to someone in need and make his or her life better.

Be big enough to reach out and lift up someone when you see he or she is down or has a burdened heart. Do this because you have deepened your sense of responsibility and obligation to demonstrate the power of God's love.

QUESTIONS FOR REFLECTION

- In the 6th commandment we learn that we're to see to it that we cause not one hardship or suffering, whatsoever. In what way do you uphold this commandment?

- What is being done at your school or college to stop bullying behavior and hate crimes? What else do you think needs to be done?

- Because to God each life has eternal value, do we have an *obligation* to carry the message of God's love to the "ends of the earth"?

- In God's eyes, what is the difference between "*murder*" and "*kill*"? In what ways do you differentiate these two?

- Do you think that the term "murderer" applies to someone who produces, sells, or advertises cigarettes or liquor?

- Do you feel that suicide is a sin? What if a person has an incurable disease or a terminal illness—might that be grounds for ending one's own suffering?

- Do you believe it is a Christian's privilege and duty to take an active interest in the civic affairs of his community and country? In what ways do you see yourself as doing this?

9

THE SEVENTH COMMANDMENT

You shall not commit adultery.

Exod. 20:14

In the previous chapter, you learned that we each are God's creation and that, as such, our lives belong to God. Because each human life has eternal value to God, He decreed human life as sacred and warned that we were not to destroy the life of another. In fact, in His very comprehensive sixth law, God also commanded that we do no bodily harm nor cause any suffering. Instead, we are to help and befriend each other in every need.

In the seventh Commandment, God expands upon how we are to conduct ourselves in relationship to others, this time as it relates to sexuality. The seventh law explicitly commands that sexual intimacy be regarded as sacred. In Genesis 2:18, we learn, "It is not good for the man to be alone; I will make a helper suitable for him." God created us to stand together, and so He joined them in marriage. Marriage, then, was a gift from God to us. God intended that marriage and family should be one of mankind's greatest joys on Earth, a foundation for true happiness.

As you already know, in each Commandment God guards something that is of the greatest importance to our welfare. What could be more basic to the welfare of a happy marriage than keeping it together? As always, there are consequences for all our actions, good or bad. God says this about anyone who should interfere with

His intention that marriage be chaste and pure between a couple: "Marriage should be honored by all . . . for God will judge the adulterer and all the sexually immoral" (Heb. 13:4). Obeying this Commandment shows that we revere, love and trust God, and love our "neighbors" as God loves us.

GOD'S SEVENTH COMMANDMENT IS STILL RELEVANT TODAY

"Pure and chaste": Does that sound old-fashioned, or what? How can this age-old Commandment possibly speak to our lives today?

It is understandable why God was concerned about the institution of marriage in times of old. It was by God's design that each man has only one wife (monogamy). But then polygamy (having two or more wives) came into existence (as a result of the falling away from God—a practice that Genesis 4:23 tells us started among the descendants of Cain). While Noah and his sons each had only one wife, polygamy crept in again, and at the time of Abraham it had become standard practice once more. At the time of Jesus, monogamy had been established among the Jews.

Why Does God Ask Us to "Hold Out" on Sex?

You are probably not marriage-minded right now. You may be in seventh grade, tenth grade, twelfth grade or college. Maybe your college years are behind you, and you are now in the workforce, or maybe you went to work full-time right out of high school. Whatever your circumstances, does this Commandment speak to you?

From the 7th Commandment we learn that God calls sex outside of marriage "adultery." If the notion of saving sex for marriage sounds old-fashioned to you, keep in mind that marriage is so esteemed by the Creator that He used the image of a bridegroom and his bride to describe the relationship between Christ and his church. In the Bible the entire "The Song of Solomon" is devoted to the beauty of married love—and discover young adults aren't the only ones who can write sizzling poems and letters about love!

God asks us to reserve sex for marriage—and to wait expectantly until the person He has ordained for us is truly ours.

"SECOND-TIME VIRGINITY"

What if you've lost your virginity and now regret that you didn't wait? Whether premarital sex was a choice you made or forced upon you, you can feel whole again. A healing release comes through forgiveness. This is important because unresolved guilt or pain kills our happiness and can even make us sick or cause depression.

Forgiving ourselves is often the hardest type of absolution. This is another reason why reading Scripture is so important. The Bible is filled with accounts that help us understand our own situation and see that God is familiar with our plight. Do you remember when the Pharisees brought a woman to Jesus whom they had caught in the act of adultery? They wanted to stone her according to Jewish law, but Jesus said, "If any one of you is without sin, let him be the first to throw a stone at her." Because they then understood, the accusers began to drift away from the scene. When they had all gone, Jesus said to the woman, "Then neither do I condemn you. Go now and leave your life of sin" (John 8:7, 11). Jesus would say to you, too, "I don't condemn you for what you've done or for what has happened to you. Go now, but sin no more." God wants you to know it's never too late to turn your life around. As we learn in Joel 2:25, "I will repay you for the years the locusts have eaten."

How? You begin by asking God to help you to once again be "chaste and pure." Reclaiming your purity can give you a whole new outlook and freedom in your life, or as we learn in 2 Corinthians 5:17, "If anyone is in Christ, he is a new creation; the old has gone, the new has come!"

While it can sometimes be very difficult for a young person to tell an adult they need help and support, especially in times like this, reach out to someone you know will listen, and help you.

God's Criteria for Finding the "Perfect" Relationship

Maybe you have a boy- or girlfriend, or maybe that's still a "to-be" for you. You never should feel pressured to be in a relationship, no matter what your age. Maybe you've decided to just focus on school, friends and sports for now, and that's good, too. Maybe you're seventeen, eighteen, nineteen or in your early twenties and already are "promised" or even engaged to someone. Maybe you're "in love" and both of you feel this way about each other, even though you know this probably isn't the person you'll marry. Or maybe it is; you've found your "one and only"—and are positive you will marry one day.

How can you be sure this person is right for you? Again, the Bible provides answers. Looking out for our relationship happiness, God laid out a blueprint for the ideal marriage in His Word. Even though you aren't married, God's plan for happiness in married life contains some good advice for making even a dating relationship a godly experience.

WHAT DOES IT MEAN TO BE "EQUALLY YOKED"?

My mother always used a phrase: "Be careful who you date: you may be choosing your mate." In my teen years, that didn't seem all that important to me, but I can see now that it really is. Choosing a "suitable" dating mate is a good thing—and it's God's desire for us, too.

He wants us to be "equally yoked." Scripture says, "Do not be yoked together with unbelievers. For what do righteousness and wickedness have in common? Or what fellowship can light have with darkness?" (2 Cor. 6:14). Being equally yoked would be a tremendous joy and blessing for the two of you.

"Equally yoked" means that the two of you agree on some very important things, the first being that you put your faith at the center of your lives. What could be more important to a couple than to share the same love of God? If both of you put God's laws first, you would be more likely to support each other in upholding the laws that God set forth to guard your well-being.

My parents divorced when I was nine. I'd like to create a home and keep it together, for always. My feeling is that if I start with being equally yoked, I'll have a better chance at that. If choosing a suitable mate is important to married life, then why wouldn't the same apply to dating life? —Chad Jarvie, 18

How can you, a young person do this? Short of going up and asking, "You're very cute; do you believe in God?", chose to be with someone who is kind and considerate, and who treats you and your friends—and his or her friends and family—with utmost respect. Know your mind and speak your mind. You don't have to "prove" anything to other friends who may want to know how far you will go.

God Knows What Makes Us Happy

You will almost surely fall in and out of love several times before you find the person who is right for you. When you make that commitment, it is intended to be for life. The Genesis story so beautifully tells of the first woman literally coming from man, *"bone of my bones and flesh of my flesh . . . For this reason, a man will leave his father and mother and be united to his wife, and they will become one flesh"* (Gen. 2:23–24). Marriage is a sacred covenant. If you and your partner are "equally yoked," meaning you share the same faith in God and enough similar interests, your relationship can be as blessed as God intended.

God's seventh Commandment is still necessary in today's times. The world might try to dismiss it, explain it away or tell us it's outdated, but it's not so. God knows what makes us happy; He knows what harms us spiritually, emotionally and physically. Misuse of sex can do all three. Maybe you know first-hand how adultery caused pain and a couple divorced after one was unfaithful to the other. Maybe you have experienced sex prematurely and have come to realize that, outside the context of marriage, it's a lot of pressure and responsibility. Remember Jesus' precious words, "Neither do I condemn you. Go and sin no more."

QUESTIONS FOR REFLECTION

- Do you and your friends discuss issues that pertain to sex, such as the consequences of unprotected sex or saving sex for marriage?

- The Song of Solomon is devoted to the beauty of love. If you haven't read it, do that now. How does the Book of Solomon "speak" to you?

- God says that we are "to wait expectantly" for the person He has "ordained" for us. What does that mean to you? Do you believe God has someone special in mind for you to love?

- What does being "equally yoked" mean to you?

- Have you ever had a boy- or girlfriend who put God first in his or her life? What was that like? Did it help you address issues such as how you should conduct yourself in the relationship?

- Do you trust God to bring the right person into your life? How will you know when that person has arrived? What are the qualities you'd like this person to have?

10

THE EIGHTH COMMANDMENT

You shall not steal.

Exod. 20:15

In the previous chapter, you learned the seventh Commandment explicitly commands that sexual intimacy be regarded as sacred—saved for marriage, privileged only for a husband and wife. Regardless of the ever-present temptations enticing our hormones, we're expected to save sex for marriage, and we're explicitly cautioned against leading others astray.

An up-close look at the eighth Commandment shows that it, too, governs personal conduct, but this time as it relates to the "property" of others. We are not to rob our fellow "travelers" of their belongings through unfair dealings, fraud or any other means.

As always, God is most sincere that we uphold His law: "[Neither] thieves nor the greedy nor drunkards nor slanderers nor swindlers will inherit the kingdom of God" (1 Cor. 6:10). Because we revere, love and trust God, and love our "neighbors" as God loves us, we uphold God's eighth Law.

IS GOD'S EIGHTH COMMANDMENT STILL RELEVANT TODAY?

As you reflect on this Commandment, assess its implications for your life. As Baron Ruzgar admitted, "God's got me on this one: There was that candy bar I stole from my neighborhood grocery store when I was eleven and the Tommy Hilfiger cap I borrowed a few months ago from Mike Olaf that I didn't return because I really like it. I sometimes take a little money from Mom's wallet without asking, and sometimes I drive the family car without permission even though I'm supposed to ask first." According to the eighth Commandment, is Baron is "guilty"?

It's not so difficult to see how Baron's taking the candy bar and the money qualify as "theft." But taking the family car without permission or the Tommy cap still hanging in his closet—did he "steal" these things, or do they fall under the category of deception? In the eyes of God, is there a difference?

HOW DOES GOD DEFINE "PROPERTY"?

For starters, "The earth is the Lord's and everything in it," we learn in 1 Corinthians 10:26.

As you know, in all His Commandments God guards something that is of great importance to our welfare. Let's have a closer look at the love behind this very important Commandment.

Is Skipping Class (or Work), Stealing?

There are many ways to take "property" from another. Stealing, robbing, cheating and deception are but a few. God says that even those who "cater to the weakness" in others are guilty of "stealing." Does this mean that someone who sells merchandise known to be harmful, such as alcohol, cigarettes or illegal drugs, is breaking God's eighth Commandment?

What about skipping class or calling in sick for school or work when you just want the day off? What about "loafing" on the job, or wasting your time and talents? Yes, all are transgressions against God's eighth Commandment.

What Belongs to God? His "These are Mine: Don't Steal Them from Me" Inventory

We transgress the eighth Commandment by withholding from God what is His. What, then, is God's? For starters, our lives, time, talent, service and love all belong to God. If we discover that we've been guilty of stealing from God—even if it's unknowingly—what should we do? According to God's Word, "He who has been stealing must steal no longer" (Eph. 4:28).

Following is a partial list of God's "property"—and God's intent for the way we should use them while on our life's journey. As you'll discover, just as we must take utmost care not to damage something we've borrowed from someone, we must be just as careful with those things on loan to us from God.

1. ***Our lives.*** Because we are all God's children, naturally we all belong to Him. He decides when we are born and when it is time for our souls to depart from their physical forms (death). Never is this more poignantly stated than in Isaiah 43:1: "I have summoned you by name; you are mine!"

    As inclusive as this is—that our very souls belong to God— we are reminded that everything we "have" and all that we are about is God's, too. This includes our time and talents, the way we treat His children (our family and friends and neighbors)— everything! The land we buy (or hope to buy) on which to build a home, our children and our children's children, the material possession we acquire—from the jewels we unearth to the fruits of our labor, all belong to God. Whatever the number of years of life we are given, we are but stewards here on Earth. As we learn in 1 Timothy 6:7, "For we brought nothing into the world, and we can take nothing out of it."

2. ***The purpose of our lives.*** "For I know the plans I have for you," declares the Lord, "plans to prosper you . . . plans to give you hope and a future" (Jer. 29:11). God assures each one of us that He has a plan for us, and so there is a purpose to our lives—and God lays claim to it. Although God expects you to "desire" wanting to find it—you are to search for it—He lets you know when you've found it. If you doubt this, ask any born-again Christian if he or she has found his or her purpose. You'll discover that this person can articulate his or her purpose succinctly, and with a great deal of zest, zeal and delight.

    Have you discovered your purpose in life? Finding it seems elusive and difficult at times, and feelings of being "empty" and "lost" are but the half of it. Solomon reminds us time and again in both the book of Proverbs and in Ecclesiastes how empty our lives can be when we focus on the wrong things. What really counts? At times when you feel maybe you haven't a clue as to what direction you should take, what sort of love, friends, career or work toward which you should be heading, have you considered that it might be God's plan that you feel a little "lost" searching on your own? God wants you to come to Him in prayer, asking Him if He'll guide you, direct you and let you know when you're on track. We shouldn't think we're to find our life's purpose on our own.

We are to ask God what He would have us do with our lives. "Teach me to do your will, for you are my God" we learn in Psalms 143:10. Have you talked to God about His intentions for your life? Have you asked God to give you insight and direction for finding your path, your work, or for simply making your way in life? He wants you to. God promises that He will put you in fertile soil where you will bloom, and that you will be like that tree planted by the water "which yields its fruit in season and whose leaf does not wither" (Ps. 1:3).

3. **The time we are given.** We are not to squander years waiting to "get a life." God gives each of us the same twenty-four hours in every day. Does God care how we spend ours? He does. At the end of time, we each will have to answer for how we spent our time on our earthly journey. It doesn't do much good to fret over someone else's life. Answering for our own is a big enough load to carry.

Have you thought about how you're going to honor God with the time He's given you? Are you using your time wisely? Have you asked Him if He's pleased with the way you're using yours? Certainly, He has much to say on this: "Sow your seed in the morning and at evening let not your hands be idle, for you do not know which will succeed, whether this or that, or whether both will do equally well. . . . So then banish anxiety from your heart and cast off the troubles of your body, for youth and vigor are meaningless" (Eccles. 11:6, 10).

How does God want you to spend your time in the future? When you think of "time," do your thoughts immediately turn to "work" or "job"? Maybe God wants you to spend your time caring for people—such as raising a family or being in a job where you tend to others, such as being a therapist. Or maybe you're to work outdoors in nature, caring for the seeds of the Earth—such as being a gardener, a farmer or working in a greenhouse. Maybe He'll ask you to build a major corporation with branches and affiliates around the world that employs thousands of people. Maybe His plan is to have you write a book that will impact the world, changing the lives of millions—or maybe it will change just one—you. Or maybe you are to be the "love" in someone's life, the ray of light and joy that gives that person strength, hope and courage to go about his or her work, a work that is destined. Who is to know? God knows. "Seek first His kingdom and His righteousness and all these things will be given to you" (Matt. 6:33). Ask God to show you His plans that will lead you to living with purpose, and hence, acquire great joy and satisfaction.

4. ***A tenth of all we earn.*** We are to consider the practice of tithing as a holy act. Because everything we have ultimately comes from God, we're honored to tithe. Does God expect us to tithe? Yes, we are to give back to God a tenth of what we earn. "A tithe of everything from the land . . . belongs to the Lord; it is holy to the Lord. Every tenth animal that passes under the shepherd's rod will be holy to the Lord" (Lev. 27:30, 32). In Genesis 28:22, we find Jacob, Abraham's grandson, pledging to God, "Of all that You give me, I will give You a tenth." And what if we skip this part of Christian living—is that okay? No. We are expected to tithe.

In fact, God considers that we are robbing from Him when we do not tithe, as we learn in Malachi 3:8: "Will a man rob God? Yet you rob Me. But you ask, 'How do we rob You?' In tithes and offerings" (Mal. 3:8). God accepts more than just our money as a tithe. As an example, our "time" belongs to God, yet He gives us the free will to spend our time as we choose—although He did set aside Sundays for us to give back to Him. Our service to God or in the church is both a time and a talent tithe, then. Still, it's only one way we're to tithe. God's ultimate intention for our tithe is that it be used to further His Word to spread the message of Jesus. And by the way, God bestows blessings on those who tithe.

Does God expect us to be prosperous, then? While God does not speak to the standard of living to which we are to aspire, the eighth Commandment carries a warning about laziness ("slothfulness"). Laziness is covered many times in the book of Proverbs and elsewhere in the Bible. We are to earn our way. Not doing so is another form of theft. "If a man will not work, he shall not eat" (2 Thess. 3:10). We are to value work. Adam and Eve had work to do even before they totally goofed up the paradise plan (Gen. 2:15). God especially admonishes us to keep out of debt. "Let no debt remain outstanding except the continuing debt to love one another" (Rom. 13:8). We are to pay our way and to pay our debts. God expects us to be prudent, and to neither squander nor waste. "Gather the pieces that are left over. Let nothing be wasted" (John 6:12).

5. ***Our fellowship (relationships) to others.*** Because we are all God's "children," we naturally should desire to help one another. In Matthew 10:42, we learn about the simple art of sharing: You don't have to do more than give "even a cup of cold water" in Jesus' name to be of service. It pleases God to see us serving others and following the example that Jesus set for us when he walked the Earth. Not only is our "caretaking" of each other commanded but doing so is good for our health and well-being. It's a well-known fact that one of the best prescriptions for feeling down is to help a person in need. Start by giving a happy heart and a joyous spirit to others in your day-to-day living.

The gift of fellowship means that we are to look out for each other—to be our "brother's keeper." We must all commit to dealing fairly, to being honest, and to working for social conditions that make it possible for all to live in abundance in all the ways we can.

6. ***Our talents and innate gifts.*** Gifts and talents are those special abilities that we each are given. Sometimes we refer to these as "our strengths." Even though some people believe they have no special talent or gift, we each receive something. While for some this may be the gift of an outgoing and engaging personality, for another it may be the gift of a serene and peaceful nature. "To one there is given through the Spirit the

message of wisdom, to another the message of knowledge by means of the same Spirit, to another faith . . . to another gifts of healing . . ." (1 Cor. 12:8–9). Yes, we've each been blessed with an attribute or strength that can be given back to God.

Our gifts, talents and special abilities are to be used in service to our "brothers and sisters" in the world. We're to reach out to others, to witness God's love and to share the Word of God. We're to serve those with whom we share our lives, and those whom God places in our path throughout the course of our lives. Why are we to do this? Because we hear God when He tells us that He wants us to love each other, as He so loves us. We are to do all we can to see to it that each hears the Word of God.

Why didn't God just give us all the same talents? These, too—our differences—are gifts from God. We each see and hear and learn things differently. What have you learned about yourself? Have you discovered, for example, that you best learn by hearing about something, or do you learn something more easily when you see it demonstrated? Maybe visual images best "speak" to you, or maybe it is through the power of music. These differences are much needed, as we learn in Ephesians 4:12–13. Blend your gifts together "so that the body of Christ may be built up until we all reach unity in the faith and in the knowledge of the Son of God and become mature."

Protecting God's Abundance

We learn that the eighth Commandment is not just about taking possessions from our neighbor. It is also about understanding what belongs to God. It's about being grateful for our lives and all that we have. It is about pulling our own weight, taking responsibility for the quality of our lives, while always remembering that we live in concert with others. We learn that the most grand of all goals we set and achieve is that we be "good and faithful servants" to our Heavenly Father, our Creator. We learn that tithing is to thank God for our abundance, so He will continue to bless us abundantly. It is about spreading the "Good News" to those with whom we share our time on Earth, as well as to those who come behind us.

By using the talents, gifts and nature of our personalities, we come to learn how each of us is needed—the different ways each of us is "called" to do God's work. In order to revere, love and trust God, and love our "neighbors" as God loves us, we must see that all our "brothers and sisters" are cared for, wherever they may call home on the planet. The apostle Paul writes, "We are God's fellow workers" (1 Cor. 3:9).

QUESTIONS FOR REFLECTION

- How does God define "property"?

- In God's eyes, what is "stealing"?

- Do you think that someone who sells merchandise known to be harmful—such as alcohol, cigarettes or illegal drugs—is breaking God's eighth Commandment?

- In what ways are acts such as skipping class, or wasting your time and talent considered stealing?

- Have you discovered your "purpose" in life? Have you talked to God about His intentions for your life? Have you asked God to give you insight and direction for finding your path, your work and your way in life?

- What strengths, gifts and talents have been given to you by God?

- God's Word admonishes us to keep out of debt. Why do you think that staying out of debt is important to God?

- What do you think this Scripture means? "Do not let the sun go down while you are still angry" (Eph. 4:26).

- In what ways would the world be different if everyone upheld God's eighth Commandment?

11

THE NINTH COMMANDMENT

You shall not give false testimony against your neighbor.

Exod. 20:16

By now you've come to see that God keeps a vigilant eye on all His creation. His house rules are straightforward: We are to revere, love and trust in God, and love each other as He loves us.

As in all His Commandments, God guards something that is of the greatest importance to our welfare. In the eighth Commandment, God focused on theft. Because we all are His children, God rightly warned us that taking or stealing the "property" of another also was a theft against Him. In this chapter, the study of the ninth Commandment, God informs us that a "good name" is also an asset—one that is so highly prized, so valuable to each of us, that in no way are we to "steal it." We are not to tarnish, diminish or slander our neighbor's name. God is specific in what He means by this: We should not lie to, betray, slander or criticize our neighbor. In this Commandment, God says of our neighbor that we are to "apologize for him, speak well of him and put the most 'charitable construction'" on all he or she does.

Our Heavenly Father is serious about our understanding and abiding by His law: "A good name is more desirable than great riches" (Prov. 22:1). Because we revere, love and trust God, and love our "neighbors" as God loves us, we consider it our honor, as much as it is our obligation, to hold our neighbor's name and reputation in the highest regard, knowing how important it is to his or her welfare.

God's Ninth Commandment Is Still Relevant Today

In days of old, much like now, a person's reputation was most important. Whether accurate or not, others judge us—and hence treat us—according to our reputation. One can only speculate how this played out in biblical days, although surely if one had a reputation for being less than upright, it wasn't like you could hire a team of forensic specialists to see you through an ordeal. A reputation could work in your favor, as well, such as in the Good Samaritan story found in Luke 10:30–37.

Whether you're called a thief or a Good Samaritan, your reputation walks into the room before you do. God rightly warns us that we are not to go around "dissing" others. We're to make sure that any negative connotation associated with someone's name not be of our own doing, nor a by-product of words we let roll off our tongues. We're to speak only of the good we know about others, and, in fact, we're charged with putting the most "charitable construction'" on all that our neighbor does. Who does God consider to be our neighbor, and what does God consider to be a violation of His "giving false testimony" law?

Who Is Our "Neighbor"?

Silly question? Not really. Yes, it is the people who live in the house next door to you, of course, but in a larger sense, it includes others. For starters, it includes everyone with whom you come in contact daily. Every person in the world is your neighbor.

There is no one in the world who is not your neighbor. As you would suspect, God's ninth Commandment applies to all His people. From the members of your family to your closest friends, from far-off countries, all are your "neighbors."

What Does "Giving False Testimony" Mean?

What does it mean to give false testimony against your neighbor? God doesn't mince words: We should not lie to, betray, slander or criticize our neighbor. We are responsible to God for the ways we uphold—or corrupt—the good name of others. Words, we learn, are deeds. "Do not let any unwholesome talk come out of your mouths, but only what is helpful for building others up according to their needs, that it may benefit those who listen" (Eph. 4:29). We are not to use our words to inflict hurt, pain or embarrassment upon anyone. Nor are we to use words that are meant to deceive, disparage or diminish the joyous and happy nature of our neighbor. The adage, "Sticks and stones may break my bones, but words will never hurt me," is not true. Words carried on the wings of love can soothe, heal, bring joy and possibility, while words riding the waves of anger leave destruction, pain, heartache and despair in their wake.

Giving false testimony results in loss. Damaging one's good name has ramifications, such as a tarnished reputation. We must not do this to our neighbor, but instead, guard our neighbor's name: "Each of you must put off falsehood and speak truthfully to his neighbor, for we are all members of one body" (Eph. 4:25). What should we do if we hear someone else uttering false testimony against our neighbor? God is clear in His direction: We should speak up, apologize for him and put the most charitable construction (to speak well of) on all that he is. We are to follow the example of Christ, who even when crucified put a charitable construction on this vile act of His enemies. He said, "Father, forgive them, for they know not what they are doing" (Luke 23:34).

The Value of a "Good Name"

What, then, we might ask, is the worth of a good name—and how destructive is a poor reputation? God leaves little doubt as to the importance of our "good name." The Bible tells us a good name is part of our daily bread. A good reputation has to do with making our way in life, whether it be to gain friendship or earn a living. Everyday experiences tell us people are unwilling to employ a person who has a reputation for being dishonest or unreliable.

On the other hand, many are chosen for positions of trust and responsibility purely on their reputations for honesty and dependability, as sixteen-year-old Holly Stinson, who works part-time at a department store, found out.

> *A girl in my department had been with the company longer than any of the other full-time employees, so she was in line for a promotion to assistant manager. Still, she didn't get the job. It was given instead to a girl with the least amount of time on the job, all because everyone spoke well of her, always saying how impeccably honest she was and what a wonderful way she had with customers. Everyone knows that it was her reputation as a "wonderful employee" that won her the job.* —Holly Stinson, 16

How have you seen the worth of a good reputation in your role as a student? A lot of grading is subjective, and teachers tend to give the benefit of the doubt to students known for their commitment to their studies. On the other hand, students with a reputation for not being "serious," or those who have been caught cheating on their assignments may find it affects their grades. Robbie Carlton, seventeen, recalls such an incident that happened to him, one that created a great deal of stress.

> *Chemistry is my toughest subject, and I really must work at it. I did well on it, to which the student behind me called out, "He cheated!" I didn't, but the teacher called me in and had me take the test over. Because I knew the material, I passed it, too. But on the day of our next test, the teacher moved me to the front of the room, presumably to keep an eye on me to be sure I wasn't cheating. Being singled out and asked to take a seat up front was embarrassing and demeaning. Worse, I never felt the "benefit of the doubt" from that teacher from that time forward.* —Robbie Carlton, 17

Four Ways We Give False Testimony

Eroding the name of another creates loss in one way or another. Whether it be loss of a position, reputation, opportunity or income, if we cause (or contribute to) loss, it is an act of wrongdoing in God's eyes. There are many ways we can give false testimony against our neighbor, including these four "biggies":

1. **To lie.** We give false testimony when we make statements about someone that are not true. Whether we do this to protect ourselves or someone else or feel that doing so is a way to better our situation (or someone else's), all are most displeasing to God.

   A kid at my school accused Alain of stealing money out of his backpack, but I knew Alain didn't take it—because I knew who did, and it wasn't Alain. But I didn't speak up and defend Alain, and that wasn't right. I still feel bad about it because I get upset when I'm accused of things that I don't do. —Robbie Wentzel, 12

2. **To betray.** Revealing the secrets of another or disclosing private and personal information is another way we give false testimony against our neighbor. All can result in *the loss of a "good name," as fifteen-year-old Larissa Linn knows because she did this to a teammate and saw how it all played out.*

3. **To slander.** Slander is another way we give false testimony against one another. When we make malicious comments about someone, such as spreading gossip, or even when we pass along information knowing it's going to hurt or diminish the name of someone (even though it may be true), then we are sinning against God's ninth Commandment.

4. **To criticize.** Do you know anyone who is always finding fault with someone? Always being critical, finding fault and being ungrateful are more than personality problems and character flaws. Why is criticism wrong in God's eyes? We might ask the question in this way, "What is the importance of speaking well of each other?" To help each other feel hope, to see possibility, to feel inspired to do what is good and best and right helps each of us to move toward harmony and peace

with one another. Has someone reached out when you were suffering a disappointment, nursing a broken heart or feeling overwhelmed? When we help others by sweetening life's joys and easing the bitterness of its disappointments and losses—by helping them to see our world as full of hope, less impossible and more glorious—we inspire and motivate them to be more caring, helping and loving people. If we let them know that we will be there to help them out, whatever their situation or station in life, then we can change the world just by changing that one person's life. That is what God wants for us. We are to be our brother's keeper. It is our obligation—as much as it is our honor—to help others daily to see their lives in the most positive light.

If an Attorney Defends Someone Who is Guilty, Is He or She Breaking the Ninth Commandment?

What would you do if you were in a situation in which you felt you had to tell a lie because something terrible might happen if you didn't? Galen Lenz's brother sometimes finds himself in this position. As Galen reports:

My brother is an attorney. He says in his profession, it's hard to be representing someone, believing that person is innocent, and then finding out he or she is not. As that person's advocate, he has the responsibility to represent that person, so then he must build a case for that person's innocence, knowing he or she is not. If he knows before he's taken on a person as a client that the person is guilty and looking for someone to get him off, then my brother won't take the case. —Galen Lenz

What do you think? Is Galen's brother guilty in the eyes of God? You might want to ask your parents, friends and youth pastor to talk this over with you.

Speaking God's Truths

Especially when we're young, it can seem like having the "scoop" on someone, to bring information to the table, can make you feel like you're "in the know." Always, it seems, people are willing to "get the goods" on someone—certainly our tabloids make us think so. Guard against thinking that you gain favor and power with others in this way.

Giving false testimony against anyone not only hurts that person, but tarnishes our own reputation, as well. If you are the sort of person who is the bringer of the "juicy news," then others will see you as a person who is all too happy to diss others. This reputation will be a mark on your own good character and set you up as someone who cannot be trusted. If someone talks poorly of another, do you think ill-spoken words about you are far behind? And what if you are not the person who is in the habit of treating others so poorly? You might look to Scripture to get up the courage to alert someone about the "wrong" they are doing or make the decision to leave this so-called friend behind. As we learn in 1 Corinthians 15:33, "Bad company corrupts good character."

Aside from letting each other down when we make it our business to put a mark on someone's name, an even bigger transgression is going on: We are expressly going against the Commandment that God has given us for how we are to revere, love and trust him, and love each other as He so loves us.

Start today by ensuring that everything you say and do honors the good name of others.

QUESTIONS FOR REFLECTION

- Give an example of a time when your good name was "jeopardized" and what you did to "salvage" it.

- Do you think it's important to safeguard "God's reputation"? In what ways do you do this?

- "A good name is more desirable than great riches" (Prov. 22:1). What does this Scripture mean to you?

- Do you believe that words, like actions, are deeds?

- We are told not to use words that deceive, disparage, disrupt or diminish the joyous and happy nature of our neighbor. What do you think this means?

- "Bad company corrupts good character" (1 Cor. 15:33). What does this Scripture mean to you?

- God leaves little doubt as to the importance of our "good name." What is the value of your "good name"? Have you ever lost your good name? What did you have to do to earn it back?

- The Bible tells us a good name is part of our daily bread. What do you think this means?

- In what ways would the world be different if everyone upheld God's ninth Commandment?

12

THE TENTH COMMANDMENT

You shalt not cover your neighbor's house. You shall not covet your neighbor's wife, or his manservant or maidservant, his ox or donkey, or anything that belongs to your neighbor.

Exod. 20:17

In the previous chapter, you learned how God considers our "good name" so valuable to each of us that He commands us not to slander, tarnish or diminish a person's reputation in any way. Not only are we not to "smear" anyone, but we're to see each other in the most positive light we can. The Bible says we're to put the most "charitable construction" on all a person does. We need to ask ourselves why we would consider it our business to do a "takeover" on someone's name—certainly a person's own words and actions can speak for themselves. If we put a mark on someone's name due to having a mean spirit, jealousy or some reason we think is justified, it's not a good thing, and we'll have to answer to God for all we say and do.

The tenth Commandment is about a "takeover" as well, this time as it relates to "coveting" that which belongs to another. "Coveting" refers not only to taking someone's possessions, but to even being desirous (jealous) of things that belong to another. The first part of the tenth Commandment deals with real estate; the second portion deals with relationships and personal property.

As in all the Commandments, God guards something that is

most important to our welfare. That we not contribute in any way toward anyone losing his or her possessions—be it that person's real estate or personal belongings, or the loyalty of that person's friends or other liaisons and associations—is certainly important to the well-being of all. Upholding the tenth Commandment shows that we revere, love and trust God, and love our neighbors as God loves us. As always, there are consequences should we not observe God's Word: "Watch out! Be on your guard against all kinds of greed; a man's life does not consist in the abundance of his possessions" (Luke 12:15).

God's Tenth Commandment Is Still Relevant Today

It's not so difficult to see why a law commanding that someone not run off with your donkey or ox or wife (in the days of Moses, even a man's wife was considered his property) was necessary in biblical times. All were vital to day-to-day existence. But that was then, and this is now. You probably don't own a donkey or ox, or even want to. You know you can't afford a mortgage just yet, and besides, maybe you don't even like the style or location of your neighbor's house. And though your neighbor may have a wife or a husband, you're quite certain you're not looking for either just yet. As for coveting your neighbor's servants, well, you're not even sure if the neighbors have household help—and besides you know how to bake a pizza and you don't even want your parents to enter your room.

While you may not want an ox or a donkey, transportation is still very much an "item." Have you ever watched as someone got out of a "to-die-for" car and wished it were in your possession? Did you ever sometimes wish you were the person who possessed such beautiful wheels (or other things)? Or maybe you wished you had his or her job or lifestyle (or parents) to be able to afford such expensive things. Have you ever coveted anything? While you may not desire someone's spouse, maybe you sometimes look at your friend's boy- or girlfriend and wish that person had "feelings" for you rather than your friend. Or you may be desirous of someone's clothes, jewelry, cell phone or other gadgets. If you ever wished a certain friend's parents were yours, or that you could be a certain movie star or maybe even just the most popular person at school, college or where you work, then you'll want to consider how any or all are viewed considering the tenth Commandment.

What Does It Mean to "Covet"?

The tenth Commandment speaks to us regarding our "wished we had" list. Coveting—desiring that which belongs to someone else, even to the point of wanting to obtain it—is an easy thing to do when we're very young. As children, we sometimes coveted our friends' toys, even to the point of reaching out and taking them and crying when we were told to give them back. It's natural for children to want to take whatever they want. But as we mature, we come to realize that such behavior is no longer acceptable, and that it is wrong to take that which belongs to another.

Why Is Coveting So Dangerous?

One reason coveting is so dangerous is because of where it can lead. When people desire the possessions of others, they may dream up a scheme to get them, steal them outright or even resort to underhanded means, such as murder, to possess them for themselves. Another reason we are not to covet the possessions of others is because such feelings can take over our hearts, separating us from God, as well as put a wedge between us and our neighbors, which you'll see is a common theme in the next section. God wants us each to earn our own way and to be grateful for what we have so as not to be consumed with desire for what others have. And yes, there is a difference between coveting and the longing for improvement and progress. The wish to improve oneself through work, study and industriousness are Christlike principles. This mind-set and work ethic go hand-in-hand with assisting and serving our neighbor.

This whole ideal is so important, so valuable, that God guards it by asking that we each look within. We each are to examine our heart to see that our motives are as pure as they can be. Your life—and all the things that you acquire—are about the abundance between you and God. God wants us to know that we can overcome temptation by asking Him to forgive us of our transgressions and to help us not to be tempted in the first place.

Coming to Terms with Greed, Envy and Jealousy— A Word from Your Peers

Here are some of the ways young people say today's world make it "almost natural" to "covet"—and how they ask God to help them change their ways.

About three months into our school year, a new girl transferred to our school from out of state. The minute I saw Penny Hill, I fell madly in love. Three days later, I saw my friend, Jeremy, standing at his locker talking to Penny. As it turned out, she was instantly goo-goo over him. I was so jealous of my friend that I started bad-mouthing him to Penny every chance I got. I'd belittle him or make him the butt of jokes right in front of her as often as I could. But Penny saw through what I was doing, and if she saw Jeremy with me, she wouldn't come up to us; she'd wait for when she could be with him when I wasn't around. That pretty much ended my hanging around with Jeremy, and worse, it put a dead halt to my being able to be anywhere near Penny. Jealousy can ruin things. I lost a dear friend, and even if Jeremy and Penny break up, there is no way she'll ever give me the time of day. Truth is, he might not either. — Jonathan Morgan, 16

My best friend, Julie Green, and I both wanted to own a car so badly. Neither of us could afford even an older one. Nor could our parents afford to help us out. Although we did get part-time jobs, we carried a heavy load of classes and neither of us could work many hours, which made saving for a car a near impossibility. Then Julie's grandparents bought a new car and gave her theirs. I was so jealous that I would make snide remarks about her having "rich relatives" which wasn't the case at all. My behavior put a strain on our relationship, but Julie was happy to give me a ride whenever she could. Still I remained jealous of her and wished that her good luck had been my own. I finally asked God to help me stop feeling jealous and simply be happy for my friend. I try to just stay in a "grateful" frame of mind; doing this makes all the difference. I feel like a better friend, and I am optimistic that I will bring the things I want into my life in time. —Joanie Fulton, 18

Greed, envy and jealousy only serve to detract us from our best intentions and derails us from healthy and straightforward relationships with family, friends and others; and keep us mired in a pettiness that consumes us, keeping us from all that is good and best about our own lives. Moreover, dwelling in the pits of such destructive emotions separates us from God.

God wants us to be grateful for what we have in our lives, so we won't be consumed with desire for what others have. This whole ideal is so important, so valuable, that God guards it by asking for each to look within. We each are to examine our hearts, to see that our motives are as pure as they can be. Your life—and all the things that you acquire—are about the abundance between you and God. Have you taken recent inventory of all you have? Have you thanked God for all He has given you? When we really look at our lives, we realize that we have so much. Decide to live your life as simply as you can. Ask God to guide you, and guard you, in your daily life. Ask Him to help you see the bigger picture—to help you understand the purpose of your life—which is to come to know God and have a personal relationship with Him. This will help you see your life as full, abundantly full. As we are reminded in Luke 12:15, "Watch out! Be on your guard against all kinds of greed; a man's life does not consist in the abundance of his possessions." There is only one thing that is worth "coveting" and that is our relationship with God: "Show me your ways, O Lord, teach me your paths; guide me in your truth and teach me, for you are God my Savior, and my hope is in you all day long" (Ps. 25:4–5).

QUESTIONS FOR REFLECTION

- Think about your lifestyle. In what ways do you break the tenth Commandment? In what ways do you uphold it?

- "Coveting" refers to not only taking others' possessions, but even to being jealous of things that belong to another. What were you jealous about? How are things now?

- How would you explain to someone that it's wrong to covet someone else's possessions?

- God wants us to be grateful for what we have so we are not consumed with desire for what others have. How do you remind yourself to be grateful for what you have?

- What is the difference between "coveting" and "wishing for improvement and progress"? Why does God approve of improving oneself through work, study and industriousness?

- In what ways would the world be different if everyone upheld God's tenth Commandment?

For You and You Alone

All the ways You work in my life are amazing, God,
And I want to thank You for taking the time;
Sins can be so heavy and disgraceful,
I'm so grateful You've forgiven me mine.

I know that at times I'm not always attuned,
And that I let the world suck the life out of me;
And I confess to getting sidetracked,
From the heir you intended me to be.

Faults or flaws—You love me nonetheless,
You're the most unconditional love of all;
On the road of life, I fail, stumble and trip,
Always You catch me the moment I fall.

God, please help me live a Christian life,
To make Your perfect will my own;
Please help me dedicate my life to You,
And live it for You, and You alone.

—Sarah Erdman, 16

New from TEEN TOWN PRESS
an Imprint of Bettie Youngs Book Publishing Co., Inc.
. . . the SMART TEENS-SMART CHOICES series
www.BettieYoungsBooks.com • info@BettieYoungsBooks.com

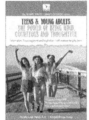

The Power of Being Kind, Courteous and Thoughtful

Information, Encouragement and Inspiration—with commentary by Teens
Jennifer Leigh Youngs, A.A. / Kendahl Brooke Youngs

- *the power of being KIND*
- *the importance of being COURTEOUS*
- *how to be "THOUGHTFUL"*

Book: 978-1-940784-82-3
e-book: 978-1-940784-83-0

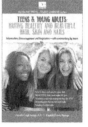

Having Healthy and Beautiful Hair, Skin and Nails

Information, Encouragement and Inspiration—with commentary by teens
Jennifer Leigh Youngs, A.A. / Kendahl Brooke Youngs

- *how to clean and care for your skin*
- *BEAUTIFUL hair; best styles for you*
- *choosing soaps and shampoos best for YOU*
- *grooming your hands, feet, and nails*

Book: 978-1-940784-84-7
e-book: 978-1-940784-85-4

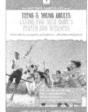

Caring for Your Body's Health and Wellness

Information, Encouragement and Inspiration—with commentary by teens
Jennifer Leigh Youngs, A.A. / Kendahl Brooke Youngs

- *food—your body's source of energy*
- *sleep—restores body and brain*
- *liking the face in the mirror*
- *stress, anxiety, and emotional ups and downs*

Book: 978-1-940784-88-5
e-book: 978-1-940784-89-2

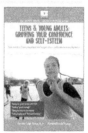

Growing Your Confidence and Self-Esteem

Information, Encouragement and Inspiration—with commentary by teens
Jennifer Leigh Youngs, A.A. / Kendahl Brooke Youngs

- *being on good terms with YOU*
- *feeling "good enough"*
- *liking the face in the mirror*
- *being happy and "forward looking"*

Book: 978-1-940784-86-1
e-book: 978-1-940784-87-8

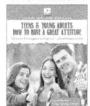

How to Have a Great Attitude

Information, Encouragement and Inspiration—with commentary by teens
Jennifer Leigh Youngs, A.A. / Kendahl Brooke Youngs

- *why attitude matters*
- *5 ways to get others to like you*
- *how to grow a terrific attitude*
- *liking the face in the mirror*

Book: 978-1-940784-90-8
e-book: 978-1-940784-91-5

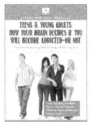

How Your Brain Decides If You Will Become Addicted—Or Not
Information and Encouragement for Teens, with Stories by Teens
Jennifer Leigh Youngs, A.A. / Kendahl Brooke Youngs

- "using," dependency and addiction
- if you or a friend can't stop using
- Withdrawal, Relapse, and Recovery
- cool ways to say "no"

Book: 978-1-940784-99-1
e-book: 978-1-940784-98-4

The 10 Commandments and the Secret Each One Guards—For You
Information and Inspiration about Faith at Work in Our lives
Bettie B. Youngs, Ph.D., Ed.D. / Jennifer Leigh Youngs, A.A.

- how the Commandments speak to you
- the secret each Commandment guards
- using your faith to guide the choices you make
- how to be confident and bold in your faith

Book: 978-1-940784-95-3
e-book: 978-1-940784-94-6

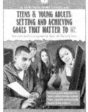

Setting and Achieving Goals that Matter to ME
Information and Encouragement for Teens, with Stories by Teens
Jennifer Leigh Youngs, A.A. / Kendahl Brooke Youngs

- discovering what's important TO ME
- hobbies, talents, interests, apptitudes
- hopes, aspirations and dreaming big
- my goal-setting workbook

Book: 978-1-940784-97-7
e-book: 978-1-940784-96-0

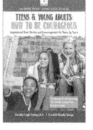

How to Be Courageous
Inspirational Short Stories and Encouragement for Teens, by Teens
Jennifer Leigh Youngs, A.A. / Kendahl Brooke Youngs

- the importance of being caring
- the benefits of being brave
- how to be a hero

Book: 978-1-940784-93-9
e-book: 978-1-940784-92-2

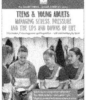

Managing Stress, Pressure, and the Ups and Downs of Life
Information, Encouragement and Inspiration—with commentary by teens
Jennifer Leigh Youngs, A.A. / Bettie J. Burres

- great ways to manage stress and pressure
- how stress works for—and against—you
- physical, emotional and behavioral signs of stress
- staying cool under pressure

Book: 978-1-940784-80-0
e-book: 978-1-940784-81-6

www.BettieYoungsBooks.com
info@BettieYoungsBooks.com

TEEN TOWN PRESS
www.TeenTownPress.com

Foreign Rights Representation: Sylvia Hayse Literary Agency, LLC
sylvia@SylviaHayseLiterary.com | C: 1.541.404.3127

Printed in the USA
CPSIA information can be obtained
at www.ICGtesting.com
LVHW091837030124
767895LV00012B/371